# The Art and Science of Thread Lifting

Bongcheol Kim · Seungmin Oh
Wonsug Jung

# The Art and Science of Thread Lifting

Based on Pinch Anatomy

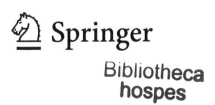

Springer

Bibliotheca
hospes

Bongcheol Kim
Lamar Clinic Isu Branch
Seoul
South Korea

Seungmin Oh
ON Clinic
Seoul
South Korea

Wonsug Jung
Department of Anatomy
Gachon University College of Medicine
Incheon
South Korea

ISBN 978-981-13-0613-6     ISBN 978-981-13-0614-3    (eBook)
https://doi.org/10.1007/978-981-13-0614-3

Library of Congress Control Number: 2018960879

This Springer imprint is published by the registered company Springer Nature Singapore Pte Ltd.
The registered company address is: 152 Beach Road, #21-01/04 Gateway East, Singapore 189721, Singapore

# Foreword

Looking back to when I first started thread lifting, it was at a point in my career when I was deeply engrossed in looking for different methods to help patients look younger. Of course, the surgical approach would be most ideal and effective, but these surgical techniques are not realistically possible to do in an aesthetic clinic. Therefore, I naturally became interested in lifting using absorbable threads.

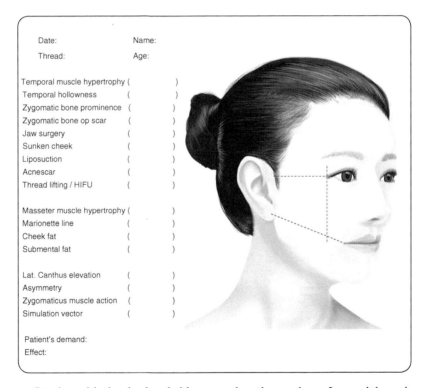

Date:                          Name:
  Thread:                        Age:

Temporal muscle hypertrophy (          )
Temporal hollowness          (          )
Zygomatic bone prominence  (          )
Zygomatic bone op scar       (          )
Jaw surgery                       (          )
Sunken cheek                    (          )
Liposuction                       (          )
Acnescar                         (          )
Thread lifting / HIFU           (          )

Masseter muscle hypertrophy (          )
Marionette line                   (          )
Cheek fat                         (          )
Submental fat                    (          )

Lat. Canthus elevation         (          )
Asymmetry                       (          )
Zygomaticus muscle action   (          )
Simulation vector               (          )

Patient's demand:
Effect:

Starting with simple absorbable mono-thread procedures, I passed through many stages of research and experience finally bringing me to this point now where I feel the need to share my journey and knowledge with the medical community.

The above figure is a chart I developed from the accumulation of my clinical and anatomical experience and knowledge which can be used to plan thread lifting procedures. Many discussions and sharing with other medical doctors have also contributed to the completion of this chart.

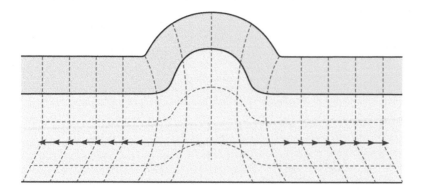

In my early years of using threads, I would attend numerous thread lifting seminars and spend the whole night pondering and working out endless questions and problems in my head. However, since threads were new and there were very little published information on them, it was very difficult to find clear evidence-based explanations to my questions. Most doctors would just say that you need to try it for yourself to find the answer.

I decided that the only choice was to experiment myself and continue to research with other colleagues to find the principles I was looking for. The above figure shows schematically the lifting mechanism of bidirectional cog threads. It depicts very simply how bidirectional cog threads can create a lifting effect.

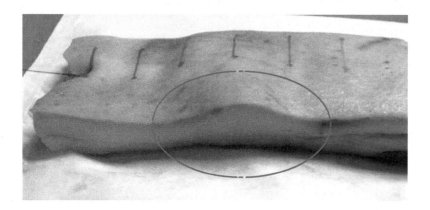

The photograph shows the lifting effects created by bidirectional cog threads in porcine tissue. As seen in the experimental porcine tissue, I tried to prove what only existed in my mind through actual experimentation. I still remember the joy of being able to physically prove the hypothetical reality and theory which existed in my mind.

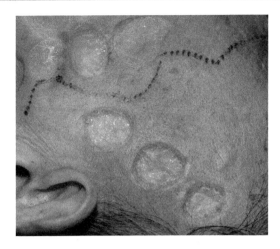

As my research accumulated one by one, the answers to 'what are the more effective and safe thread lifting methods' began to emerge.

One of them was to know how to pull the skin effectively to minimizing damage to blood vessels and nerves.

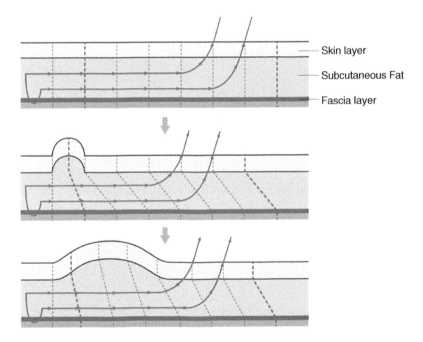

The process of compiling results and knowledge through research and experimentation studies was very difficult and challenging. However, as time passed by, these results started to form into a more organized system.

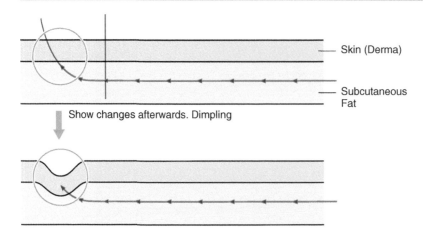

Show changes afterwards. Dimpling

It took numerous hours to write this book for the purpose of introducing safe and effective methodology to perform thread lifting. We hope that this book will serve to assist many doctors who are currently experiencing difficulties with thread lifting and who would like to perform these procedures after understanding the underlying mechanisms of thread lifting. We also sincerely hope that all doctors who read my book do not have to experience the difficulties which I had to go through to learn safe and effective thread procedures.

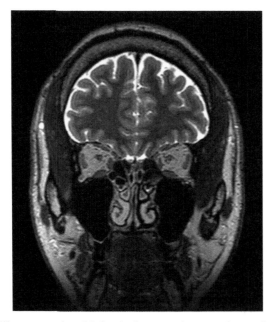

I would like to note that this book also contains experimental results of the authors and their hypotheses. These will be areas requiring further research in various fields in the future.

Through publishing this book, we also hope to make a meaningful relationship with many other doctors around the world who are interested in furthering the expertise in this field of aesthetic medicine. We also look forward to seeing more future publications which can build upon and surpass the content we have set forth here.

Seoul, South Korea                                                             Bongcheol Kim
Seoul, South Korea                                                               Seungmin Oh
Incheon, South Korea                                                             Wonsug Jung

# Note of Appreciation

Since we gathered with mutual desire of pursuing a goal of writing a book on thread lifting, several seasons have passed. Time to time, when the progress was slow and resolution could not be made, we encouraged each other to reach this place. To complete writing within a set period, we often become very tired of working restlessly. However now, we are at our final destination. Without the mutual trust in each other, we do not think we could have arrived here.

The biggest gift from writing this book may be the mutual trust in each other. Although there are remaining areas yet to be completed and to be further researched, we think that this would be helpful to those doctors who are interested in thread lifting. We would like to first thank our families who supported and encouraged us and stayed by our side as we wrote this book. Also, we are grateful to various doctors who helped us in obtaining knowledge in threads. Dr. Jihyun Lee helped us in dissection of cadavers and tissue processing. Especially, we would like to give many thanks here to Dr. Kwan Hyun Youn who completed the excellent anatomy illustrations with much effort. We promise to ourselves through this book we will continue to try with the attitude of studying continuously in the future, and we hope to contribute to brightening the bigger world for the cosmetic medicine of Korea.

Co-authors:

| | |
|---|---|
| Seoul, South Korea | Seungmin Oh |
| Seoul, South Korea | Bongcheol Kim |
| Incheon, South Korea | Wonsug Jung |

# Prior Researches

There has been inadequate high quality studies conducted on absorbable thread lifting. It is difficult to find studies that clarify the mechanism and studies regarding its effect are still in progress. Physicians inevitably have no choice but to refer to studies on non-absorbable thread lifting. Nevertheless, knowledge of facial anatomy can be applied to lifting threads regardless of its bio-absorbability.

According to Mendelson, the face is divided into the mobile frontal and the fixed lateral regions, which are separated by the vertical line from the lateral canthus. To ensure successful non-absorbable thread lifting outcomes, it is important to have a solid understanding of the distinctive characteristics of each region.

Recently, interesting results have been published from research conducted in Korea. In this study, cog and twin threads were placed and the patients were followed over a period of 24 weeks. Clinical improvement in both lifting and quality of skin texture was observed but satisfaction was higher for quality of skin texture than for lifting. The authors of the study attribute the lower satisfaction in lifting to the lack of anchoring.

Lifting effect is contingent upon anchoring. Inserting mono-threads or inserting cog threads in the subcutaneous layer and simply tugging will not yield sufficient lifting effects. For effective lifting results, a thorough understanding of fixation points is necessary. Therefore, the authors focus first and foremost on fixation points in this book.

On the other hand, there is a study that states that regardless of the plane of thread insertion, deeper tissue repositioning and augmentation is necessary to induce lifting. This is a very important point.

Analysis of structural changes with aging show that reduction in volume is a major factor in aging. Therefore, antiaging/rejuvenation treatments such as filler injections that replenish lost volume yield good clinical outcomes. These procedures are generally called "volumizing-lifting". Adding lost volume with fillers or autologous fat has the effect of shifting the deeper tissues via augmentation.

Volumizing using fillers and other materials is definitely an effective procedure. However, in patients with ptosis of skin and fat tissue due to lack of elasticity associated with aging, volumization procedures alone may not be effective. In such cases, performing volumizing procedures in conjunction with lifting procedure may result in more favorable outcomes.

To scientifically demonstrate the aforementioned clinical outcomes, the authors are planning to conduct a study called "Lifting in conjunction with volumization procedures is more effective than volumization alone."

This book also introduces case that demonstrates tissue repositioning with thread lifting via 3D scanning. The authors anticipate that a lot of research will be conducted on this subject.

After absorbable thread treatments became widespread, the authors collected patient feedback on thread lifting results. Both positive and negative comments have been received.

Below is the list of negative responses.

- The limited effect.
- Short longevity of effect.
- Possibility of severe bruising and swelling.
- Possibility of skin dimpling.
- Difficulty/inconvenience in speaking.

Efforts to address the negative responses must be made. This book contains clinical studies, experiments, and experiences that have been conducted so far. We received help from specialists in various fields, and further research is also planned.

This book addresses how to overcome the negative responses and explains how to perform effective, long lasting thread lifting procedures while avoiding complications such as swelling and skin dimpling. Complication management is also discussed.

# Author's Profile

**Bongcheol Kim**
　Director of Lamar Isu Clinic
　College of Medicine, Chonnam National University
　Internship – Samsung Medical Center (Seoul)
　Residency – Samsung Medical Center (Seoul)
　Vice president of the Korean Association for Laser, Dermatology and Trichology
　KOL of Silhouette Soft®
　KOL of QT Lift®

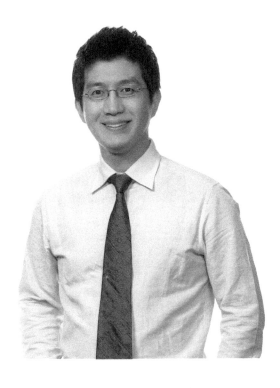

**Seungmin Oh**

Director of ON Clinic
College of Medicine, Seoul National University
Internship – Seoul National University Hospital
Residency – Seoul National University Hospital
Medical MBA, Kyung Hee University
President of OK Medi. Co,, Ltd.
Executive Board Member of the Korean Association for Laser,
Dermatology and Trichology
KOL of QT Lift®
Advisory Board Member of Hugel Co., Ltd.

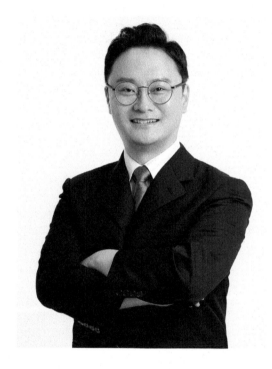

**Wonsug Jung**

Assistant Professor, Department of Anatomy, Gachon University College of Medicine

Graduated from Yonsei University College of Medicine, MD

Graduated from Yonsei University Graduate School, PhD

Member of the Korean Association of Anatomists

Member of the Korean Association of Physical Anthropologists

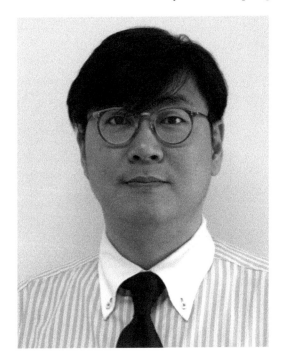

# Contents

# Part I

# Why Is Fixing Technique Important?

A successful and effective lifting treatment must be based on a thorough understanding of changes to the face due to aging. In addition, learning clear meaning of various terms used in explaining lifting is necessary.

Among the key contents used in the book, the authors obtained some of them through experiencing lifting actually. As such, if we start without clarifying the meaning of words, confusion or curiosity may occur. Accordingly, we think it is necessary to start our story after clarifying the definition and the meaning of some important terms.

## 1.1 Fixing Point

There are three important terms in absorbable thread lifting. The first one is the fixing point, the second one is the direction, and the third one is the hanging point.

As mentioned above, the concept of the fixing point is important while performing thread lifting procedure. Previous studies on the effect of thread lifting have been made without proper anchoring. This tells the reason for the poor lifting effect. A fixing point means the point which receives the pulling force when a certain part of the face is being pulled. Taking bungee jumping as an example would help to understand. Provided that jumping is done after connecting the jumping stand and the body with the rope for jumping, the jumping stand to which the rope is tied would be the fixing point.

## 1.2 Direction

Direction in lifting procedure means the vector from the hanging point to the fixing point. Direction must exist to call lifting real and a desired shape can be made. Simple thread inserting procedures without direction do not make the desired shape, whereas a lifting procedure can create a lifting effect and desired face shape with a suitable direction from the hanging point to the fixing point.

## 1.3 Hanging Point

The hanging point refers to the point at the end of the thread when the thread was inserted from the fixing point to the direction of the facial part to be pulled. In the example of pulling a sagged cheek upward, the hanging point exists at a point between the fixing point and the sagged cheek to be pulled (Fig. 1.1).

In some cases, the hanging point does not precisely coincide with the part to be lifted (Fig. 1.2). Lifting still can be possible. This is because facial tissues are intricately connected to each other by fibrotic tissues in the subcutaneous fat layer or various ligaments, etc. Especially,

© Springer Nature Singapore Pte Ltd. 2019
B. Kim et al., *The Art and Science of Thread Lifting*, https://doi.org/10.1007/978-981-13-0614-3_1

**Fig. 1.1** Definition of fixing point, hanging point, and direction. Pulling the hanging point to the direction of the fixing point is facial lifting

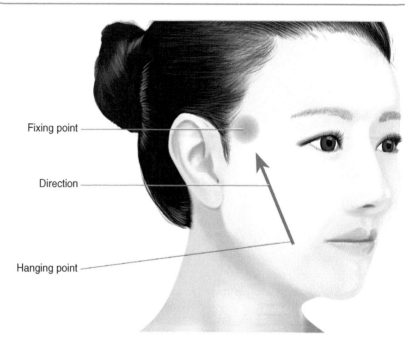

Fixing point

Direction

Hanging point

**Fig. 1.2** If the hanging point and the part to be pulled do not coincide, the actual part to be pulled is either the lower cheek or the hanging point of the thread which is the lower cheekbone. The hanging point and the part to be pulled are different

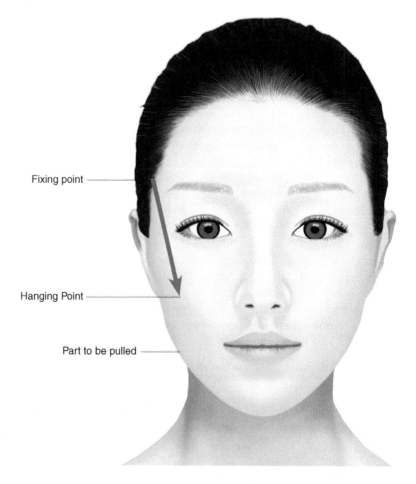

Fixing point

Hanging Point

Part to be pulled

certain areas on the face such as the lower cheek-bone area and the fibrotic tissue in the subcutaneous layer are very tough and dense. If a thread is inserted into such fibrotic tissues and pulled, these dense tissues will be pulled effectively, and tissues which are located away from the hanging point also pulled. For example, to lift the lower cheek part to the direction of the head, the thread does not necessarily have to be inserted in the lower cheek area to create a lifting effect.

However, in a certain patient group, inserting and pulling a thread only to the hard fibrotic tissue in the lower cheekbone area can bring a good effect. Therefore, patients and procedure technique selection should be well considered before treatment.

The difference between the lifting technique which can make a fixing point and the lifting technique which cannot make a fixing point is that the former clearly has direction. Various procedures which contract the skin or reduce the fat layer can make the face to appear pulled. Namely, even if there is no direction, the face can look lifted and tightened. This is related to the changes to the face as a result of aging.

As aging progresses, each plane of the face goes through changes. Various changes such as sagging of fat due to gravity, stretching of fibrotic tissues surrounding the fat, and stretching of the skin together make the aging appearance of the face.

If the skin is contracted or the fat layer is reduced, as they have effects of tightening stretched tissues, they are thought to be able to bring the similar effect of lifting. Also, through various procedures, various fibrotic tissues existing in the face can be settled and newly formed.

However, this is thought to have weaker effects than the lifting procedure which strongly forms a fixing point. The concept of the fixing point has been passed down from the past. Sulamanidze M. et al. said that thread lifting procedures consist of floating method and fixing method. Mendelson et al. classified the face into the frontal part which moves and the lateral part which is fixed.

In this regard, Hyeonho Han et al. announced that the performance of thread lifting with fixing type in the lateral part of the face and floating type in the frontal part of the face together showed good results.

The fixed type discussed here means forming a strong fixing point on the temporal fascia area. This is an important thesis discussing about the importance of the fixing point (Fig. 2.1).

To optimize lifting effects, pulling must be done with direction, and a strong fixing point must exist from the pulling direction. This is because force must support in the opposing direction from the movement of the tissues resulting from aging and gravity.

Although there is relative amount of difference in strength, each thread lifting techniques have the mechanisms of making a fixing point or roles which function the same as the fixing point. In some cases, the basis was uncovered through animal testing, and in some cases basis is not made clear. Fixing a thread in the fascia area is thought to be the strongest technique. However, this technique is not easy, and also when bleeding, the duration of the procedure takes longer, and side effects such as hematoma can possibly occur.

If knowledge can minimize the possibility of bleeding while making the fixing point strong and procedural skills are clearly made, we think that safe and effective thread lifting can be performed.

This is also the reason for talking about the fixing point first in this book. The authors performed several experiments to understand thread lifting mechanisms in the body. They will be helpful in understanding the mechanisms of thread lifting.

**Fig. 2.1** Temporal fascia. Showing the superficial temporal fascia and the deep temporal fascia. The deep temporal fascia has a part which divides into the deep layer and the superficial layer. *STF* Superficial Temporal Fascia, *DTF* Deep Temporal Fascia (Published with kind permission of © Kwan- Hyun Youn 2018. All rights reserved)

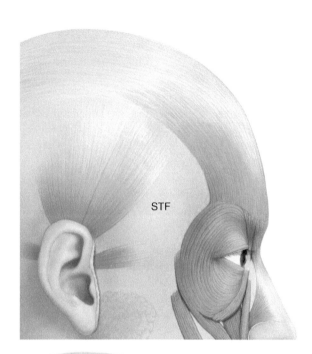

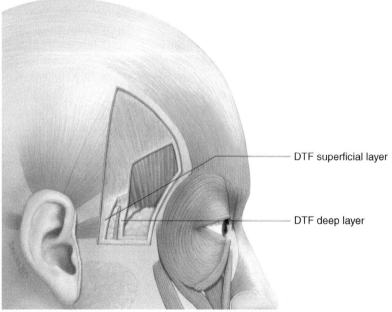

## 3.1 Method of Making a Fixing Point

The mechanism of mono-thread used in the first-generation absorbable thread lifting is expressed through this (Fig. 3.1).

Physicians expected lifting effects by inserting more threads in the direction that the face was desired to be pulled. It will be explained in the later part of this book that when the absorbable ingredient, PDO, enters into the tissue, various changes occur. Especially, changes such as contraction of tissues and proliferation of fibrotic tissues prove to some extent the theoretical basis for the thread lifting using mono-threads (Yoon JH, et al. Tissue changes over time after polydioxa-

none thread insertion: An animal study with pigs. J Cosmet Dermatol. 2018;00:1–7).

The fixing point forming mechanism is as varied as the thread lifting type. In this regard, there are not many cases which adequately explain such mechanisms. For example, they are not able to accurately explain why bi-directional cog thread or mono-thread technique causes facial lifting.

But lifting is obviously possible if the thread is hanging in a relatively firm fascia region, runs in the subcutaneous fat layer, and is then pulled. Of course, discussions about the lasting time and whether the thread really hangs in the fascia, etc. will be dealt with later. However, the lifting procedure using the method of hanging the thread in the hard fascia area and pulling is not easy to fol-

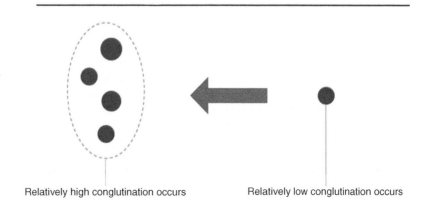

**Fig. 3.1** Forming a fixing point of monofilament threads. Formation of fibrotic tissues occurs more in the area where relatively many threads were inserted. No clear fixing point exists

Relatively high conglutination occurs

Relatively low conglutination occurs

© Springer Nature Singapore Pte Ltd. 2019
B. Kim et al., *The Art and Science of Thread Lifting*, https://doi.org/10.1007/978-981-13-0614-3_3

low due to its level of difficulty. Based on the recent trend, if there is any lifting method which can make a hard fixing point with short and simple procedure without any side effect, it would be the most ideal.

Recently, lifting is performed in the form of gathering tissues in the middle part of the thread using a bi-directional cog thread. This will be explained in the following figure, and a point which serves the similar function as a fixing point occurs in the middle part of the thread. Such method is more accurately explained as soft tissue repositioning rather than lifting.

After inserting a bi-directional cog thread and tying the threads to each other in the insertion area, the role of the fixing point can be strengthened. This is a case where the knot formed by the tie serves as a weak fixing point.

There is also a method of forming a fixing point using the hard ligament tissue in the inner side of the face. By causing the cog thread to be hung in the area of the true ligament, a hard fixing point can be formed. Places to which such special technique can be applied exist, and it can make results better than the mono-thread insertion method.

# Part II

# Facial Anatomy for Non-surgical Thread Lifting

# Anatomy for Absorbable Thread Lifting

**4**

## 4.1 Layers of the Face

Like the scalp, the facial tissue can be divided into five layers. And the face and the scalp are connected to each other layer by layer. There is an exception in the fifth layer where masticatory muscles have different embryological origins from facial expression muscles (Table 4.1 and Fig. 4.1).

### 4.1.1 Skin

In general, the skin of the male is slightly thicker than the female. And the thickness of the dermis of Koreans does not differ largely from that of Caucasians. However, the epidermis of Koreans tends to be thicker than that of Caucasians.

Table 4.2 lists the skin thickness by area based on a Korean study. It is noteworthy that the neck being the thickest among all the area measured is not a common finding in other studies. These inter-study variations probably result from the differences in the population of study and methods of measurement.

### 4.1.2 Superficial Fat

It is a layer corresponding to the hypodermis. It is located superficial to the facial expression muscles and consists of several compartments. Superficial fat sags downward by aging (Fig. 4.2).

### 4.1.3 Musculo-aponeurotic Layer/ SMAS

This layer consists of facial expression muscles and aponeurosis. And the layer is connected to the galea aponeurotica of the scalp.

Aponeurosis interconnects the platysma muscle and frontalis muscle. The aponeurosis is named differently by its relative location to the zygomatic arch; the aponeurosis upper to the zygomatic arch is being called the temporoparietal fascia or superficial temporal fascia and the part lower to the zygomatic arch the SMAS (superficial musculo-aponeurotic system).

The branches of the facial nerve innervating the facial expression muscles travel deeper than this layer, and some blood vessels (e.g., superficial temporal artery) travel within the temporoparietal fascia.

**Table 4.1** Layers of the face

|  | Facial layer | Scalp layer |
|---|---|---|
| First layer | Skin | Skin |
| Second layer | Superficial fat | Connective tissue |
| Third layer | Facial expression muscle/ SMAS (musculo-aponeurotic layer) | Aponeurosis |
| Fourth layer | Deep fat | Loose areolar tissue |
| Fifth layer | Deep fascia | Periosteum |

© Springer Nature Singapore Pte Ltd. 2019
B. Kim et al., *The Art and Science of Thread Lifting*, https://doi.org/10.1007/978-981-13-0614-3_4

**Fig. 4.1** Facial layers.
The coronal section of
the face is represented
schematically.
(Published with kind
permission of ©
Kwan-Hyun Youn 2018.
All rights reserved)

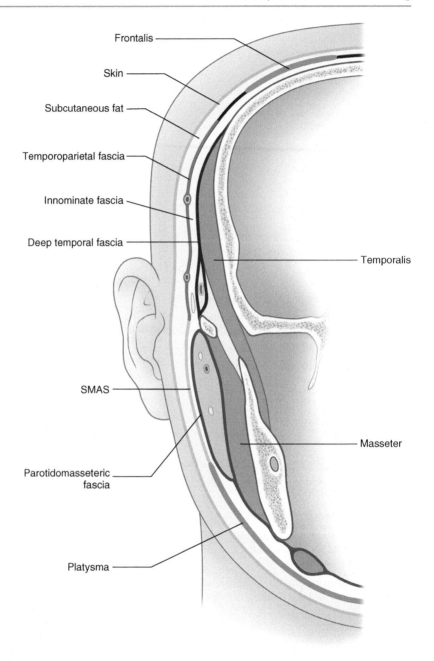

Frontalis

Skin

Subcutaneous fat

Temporoparietal fascia

Innominate fascia

Deep temporal fascia

Temporalis

SMAS

Masseter

Parotidomasseteric
fascia

Platysma

**Table 4.2** Skin thickness of Koreans

|          | Male    | Female  |
|----------|---------|---------|
| Forehead | 0.90 mm | 0.84 mm |
| Eyelid   | 0.57 mm | 0.47 mm |
| Cheek    | 1.24 mm | 1.04 mm |
| Chin     | 0.89 mm | 0.75 mm |
| Neck     | 1.56 mm | 1.26 mm |

## 4.1.4 Deep Fat

In the fourth layer of the face, there are several
spaces, and the retaining ligaments traverse
between them connecting the periosteum/deep
fascia to the skin. Deep fat is located deep to the
facial expression muscles and divided into several

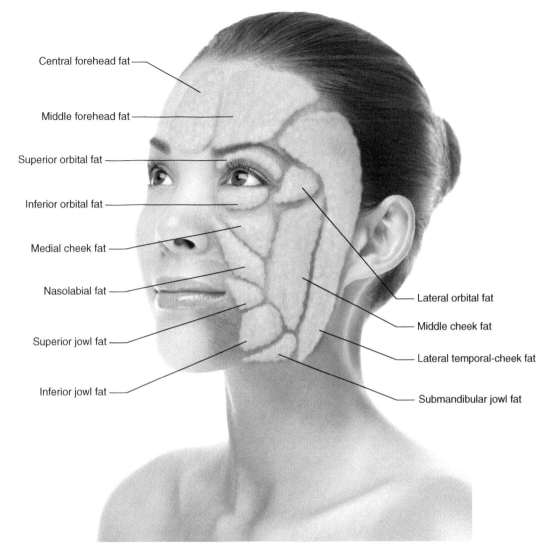

Central forehead fat

Middle forehead fat

Superior orbital fat

Inferior orbital fat

Medial cheek fat

Nasolabial fat

Superior jowl fat

Inferior jowl fat

Lateral orbital fat

Middle cheek fat

Lateral temporal-cheek fat

Submandibular jowl fat

**Fig. 4.2** Superficial fat compartments. (Published with kind permission of © Kwan- Hyun Youn 2018. All rights reserved)

compartments (Fig. 4.3). In the temporal area, the connective tissue beneath the temporoparietal fascia is called the innominate fascia.

### 4.1.5 Deep Fascia

There are masticatory muscles like temporalis m. and masseter m. in the temporal fossa and the mandible. The periosteum of the skull proceeds

as the deep fascia covering muscles of mastication (Figs. 4.1 and 4.4).

The deep fascia over the temporalis m. is called the temporalis muscle fascia or the deep temporal fascia, and it attaches to the zygomatic arch after being split into a superficial and a deep layer. There is a superficial temporal fat pad in between the two layers of the deep temporal fascia and a deep temporal fat pad which is an extension of the buccal fat pad lying

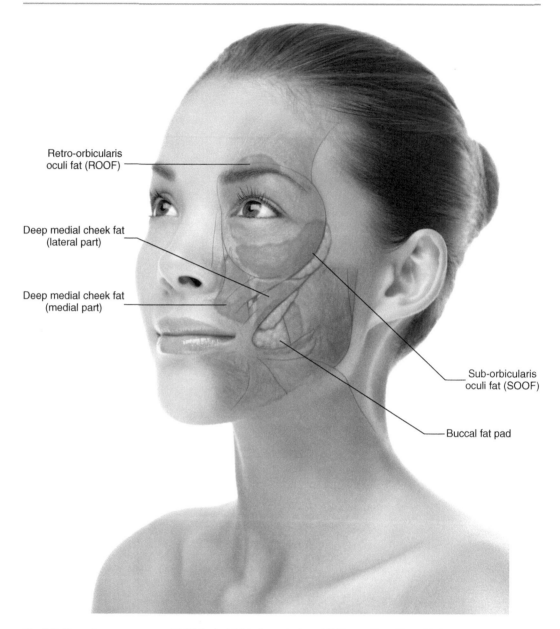

Retro-orbicularis
oculi fat (ROOF)

Deep medial cheek fat
(lateral part)

Deep medial cheek fat
(medial part)

Sub-orbicularis
oculi fat (SOOF)

Buccal fat pad

**Fig. 4.3** Deep fat compartments. (Published with kind permission of © Kwan- Hyun Youn 2018. All rights reserved)

between the temporalis m. and the deep temporal fascia.

In the mandible, the deep fascia surrounds not only the masseter m. but also the parotid gland; hence, it is called as the parotidomasseteric fascia, and it also attaches to the zygomatic arch. The musculo-aponeurotic layer/SMAS is a continuous layer, crossing over the zygomatic arch, while the deep fasciae attach to the upper and lower borders of the zygomatic arch and are not one continuous layer.

The temporal branch of the facial nerve exits the parotid gland by penetrating the parotidomasseteric fascia, and after crossing the zygomatic arch, it traverses the innominate fascia to innervate the orbicularis oculi m. and frontalis m.

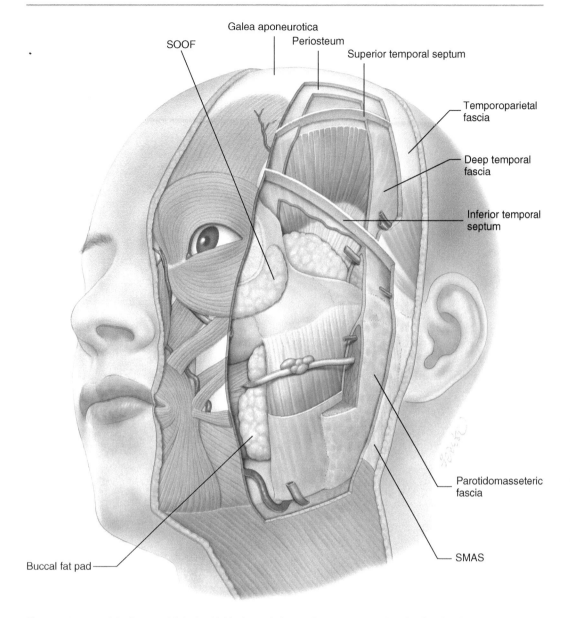

**Fig. 4.4** Layers of the face. (Published with kind permission of © Kwan- Hyun Youn 2018. All rights reserved)

## 4.2 Cadaveric Photo Series of Facial Layers

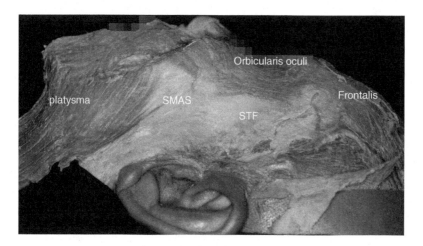

- After removing the skin and the subcutaneous fat tissues, the third layer, musculo-aponeurotic layer/SMAS, is exposed.
- Platysma, orbicularis oculi, and frontalis muscles and the interconnecting aponeurosis.
- The part of aponeurosis below the zygomatic arch is called SMAS; the part above the zygomatic arch is called the superficial temporal fascia (STF) or temporoparietal fascia.
- The musculo-aponeurotic layer/SMAS is the most important layer in the surgical lifting procedure.

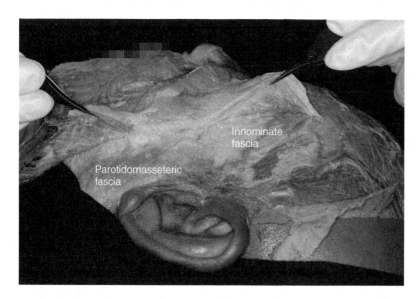

- By lifting the SMAS layer, the parotidomasseteric fascia which is the deep fascia covering the parotid gland and the fourth layer in the temporal area, the innominate fascia, are exposed.

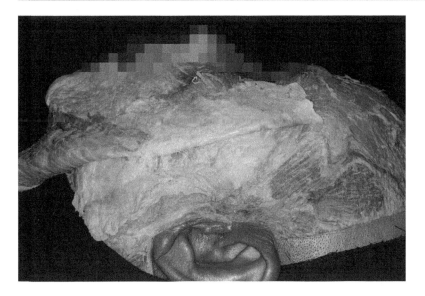

- The part of parotidomasseteric fascia covering the parotid gland is thicker than the part covering the masseter area.

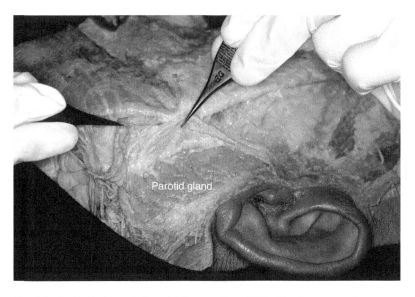

Parotid gland

- By lifting up the parotidomasseteric fascia, the parotid gland was exposed.

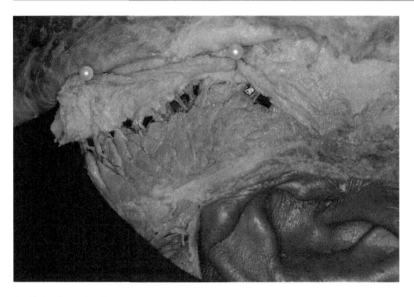

The branches of the facial nerve coming out of the borders of the parotid gland are clearly visible.

- The branches of the facial nerve travel within the parenchyma of the parotid gland.

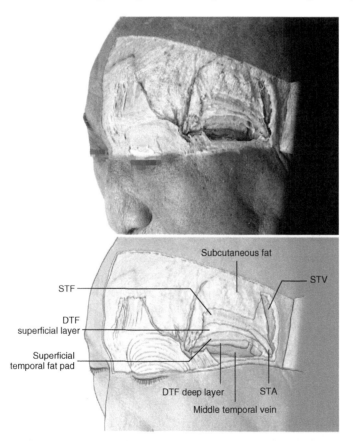

- This is a cadaveric photo showing the layers of the temple.
- The superficial temporal artery (STA) is enclosed by the superficial temporal fascia (STF).

- The middle temporal vein is embedded in the superficial temporal fat between the superficial and deep layers of the deep temporal fascia.

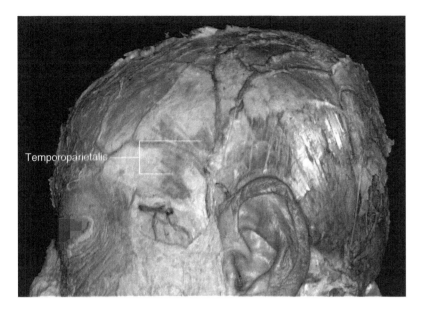

Temporoparietalis

- Note the presence of the temporoparietalis m. in the same layer as the superficial temporal fascia.

## 4.3 Anatomical Structures that Could Be Damaged During Thread Lifting

Although nonsurgical thread lifting is considered to be a minimally invasive procedure, some anatomical structures may be at risk of being damaged during treatment. Since thread lifting is performed mainly from the top to the bottom in a perpendicular direction, there is risk of injury in structures which course obliquely or horizontally in the lateral face (Fig. 4.5). Such structures are summarized in Table 4.3.

### 4.3.1 Blood Vessels

1. Frontal branch of the superficial temporal artery.

- The superficial temporary artery bifurcates into frontal and parietal branches at 18 mm anterior and 37 mm superior to the tragus.
- The frontal branch travels anterosuperiorly in the temple. It meets the lateral border of the frontalis muscle at 16 mm lateral to the lateral canthus and 15 mm above the eyebrow and then travels on the surface of the frontalis m. afterward (Fig. 4.6).

2. Zygomatico-orbital artery
- As a branch of the superficial temporal artery, the zygomatico-orbital artery exists at 80–90% and runs parallel to the upper border of zygomatic arch toward the outer corner of the eye.

3. Transverse facial artery.
- The transverse facial artery originates from the superficial temporal artery within the parotid gland and travels in the same depth as the facial nerves.
- It travels in between the zygomatic arch and the parotid gland and runs approximately 14 mm (5–26 mm) below the lower border of the zygomatic arch.

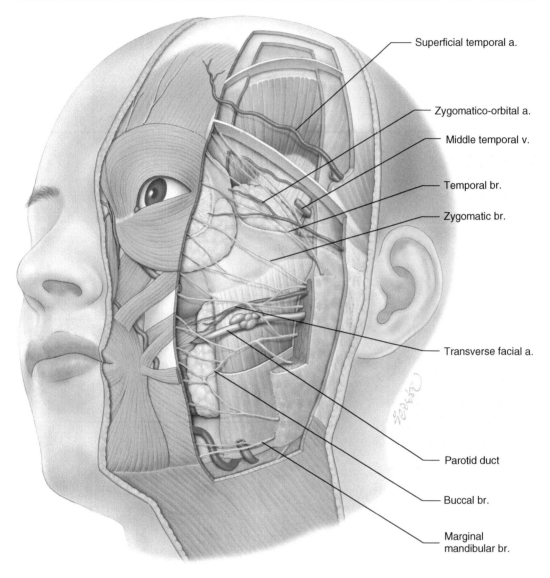

**Fig. 4.5** Anatomical structures running the lateral face horizontally or obliquely. (Published with kind permission of © Kwan- Hyun Youn 2018. All rights reserved)

**Table 4.3** Anatomical structures that could be damaged during thread lifting

| Blood vessels | Frontal branch of superficial temporal artery |
|---|---|
| | Zygomatico-orbital artery |
| | Transverse facial artery |
| | Middle temporal vein |
| Nerves | Temporal, zygomatic, buccal, and marginal mandibular branches of the facial nerves |
| Other structure | Parotid duct |

4. Middle temporal vein.
   - Middle temporal vein runs approximately 2 cm above the zygomatic arch and drains into the superficial temporal vein.
   - It runs between the superficial and deep layers of the deep temporal fascia and is embedded in the superficial temporal fat pad.

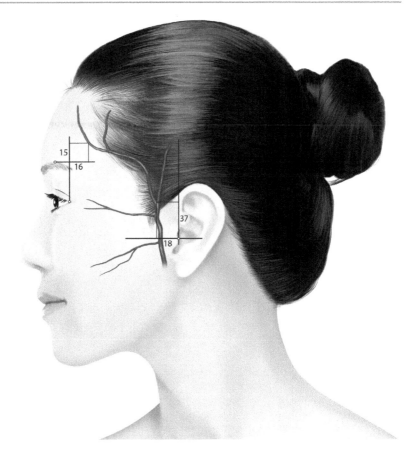

## 4.3.2    Nerves

- The temporal, zygomatic, buccal, and marginal mandibular branches of the facial nerve emerge from the parotid gland and run anteriorly beneath the SMAS.
- The temporal branch of the facial nerve exits the parotid gland by penetrating the parotidomasseteric fascia and travels up across the zygomatic arch covered by the innominate fascia. The temporal branch penetrates the innominate fascia at 1.5–3 cm above the zygomatic arch and runs just beneath the superficial temporal fascia.
- There are several temporal branches of the facial nerve, and they are located approximately within the triangle created by the earlobe, the hairline, and the lateral eyebrow.
- The temporal branch of the facial nerve courses along the Pitanguy's line which runs from a point 0.5 cm below the tragus to a point 1.5 cm above the lateral eyebrow.
- The temporal branch of the facial nerve crosses the middle third of the zygomatic arch which is 1.8 cm from the posterior end of the zygomatic arch and 2 cm from the anterior end of the arch (Fig. 4.7).

## 4.3.3    Parotid Duct

- Parotid duct generally runs above the line connecting the tragus and angle of the mouth.
- Parotid duct follows a curved trajectory from the 1/3 point and 2/3 point along the line connecting the tragus and the angle of the mouth, with the peak of curve being 1.5 cm above the line (Fig. 4.8).

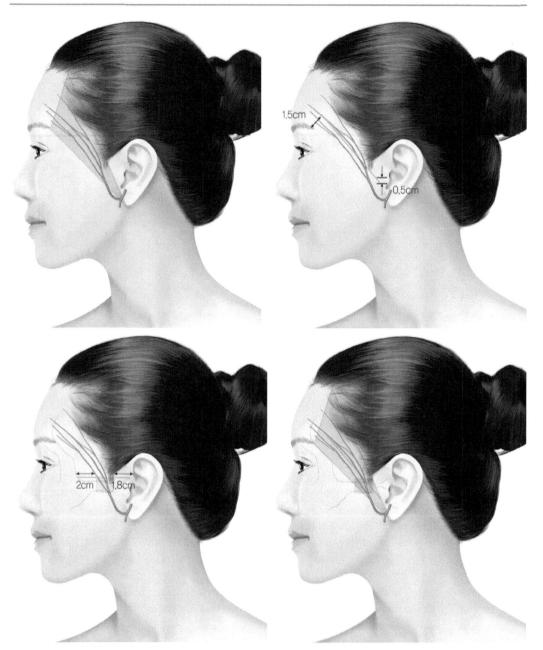

**Fig. 4.7** Pathway of the temporal branches of the facial nerve. (Published with kind permission of © Kwan- Hyun Youn 2018. All rights reserved)

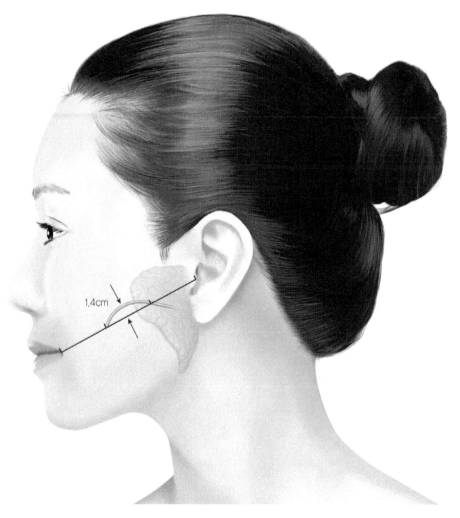

**Fig. 4.8** The course of the parotid duct. (Published with kind permission of © Kwan- Hyun Youn 2018. All rights reserved)

The photographs of the above structures are composed on a model's face (Figs. 4.9, 4.10 and 4.11) and the histologic sections containing those structures are illustrated for reference (Fig. 4.12).

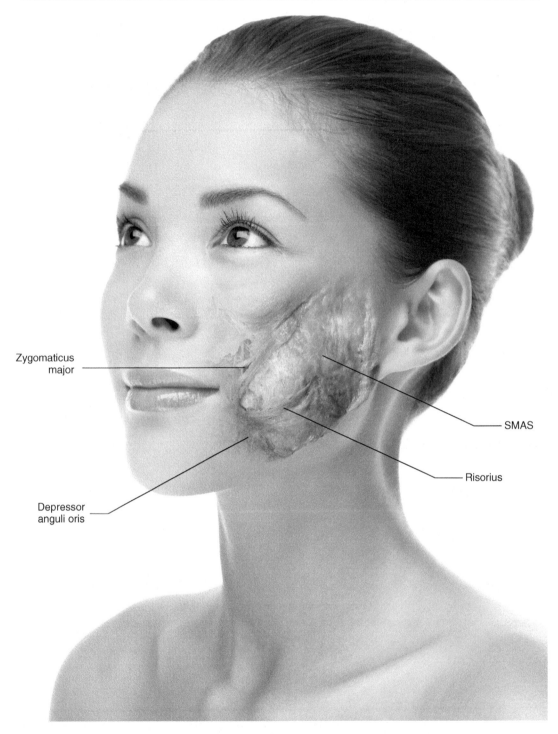

Zygomaticus major

Depressor anguli oris

SMAS

Risorius

**Fig. 4.9** Musculo-aponeurotic layer/SMAS. (Published with kind permission of © Wonsug Jung and Kwan- Hyun Youn 2018. All rights reserved)

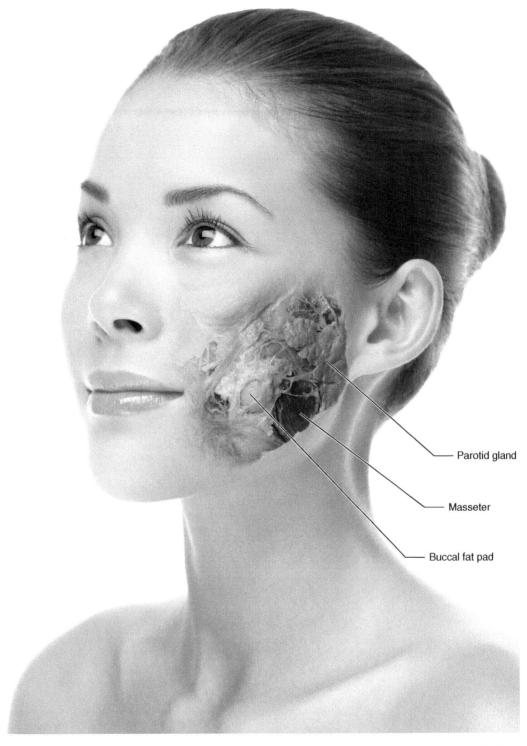

**Fig. 4.10** After removal of the SMAS and parotidomasseteric fascia, the parotid gland and branches of facial nerves exiting it can be seen. (Published with kind permission of © Wonsug Jung and Kwan- Hyun Youn 2018. All rights reserved)

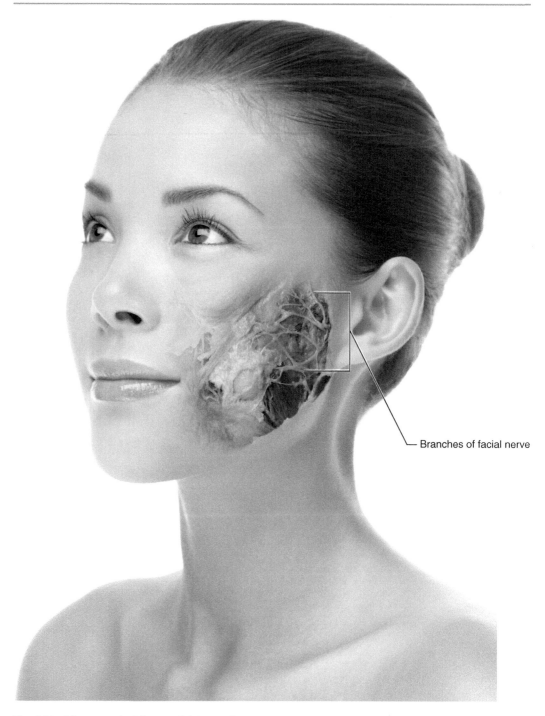

Branches of facial nerve

**Fig. 4.11** After removal of the superficial part of the parotid gland, the branching pattern of the facial nerve can be observed. (Published with kind permission of © Wonsug Jung and Kwan- Hyun Youn 2018. All rights reserved)

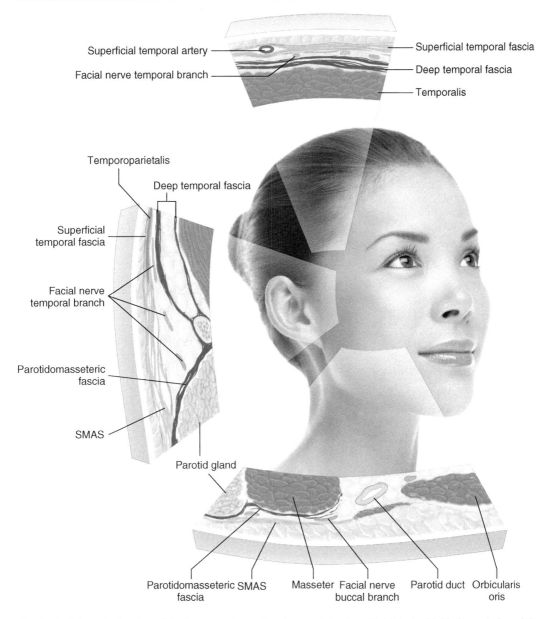

**Fig. 4.12** Schematic drawing of the tissue specimen of each area of the face. (Published with kind permission of © Wonsug Jung and Kwan- Hyun Youn 2018. All rights reserved)

# Avoiding Vessel Damages in Thread Lifting

## 5.1 Thread Lifting and Blood Vessels

Direct insertion of thread into the blood vessel does not occur easily in thread lifting, when compared to the filler injection. Therefore, vascular complications relating to thread lifting are limited to bruising, hematoma, edema, pain, etc., which are less devastating.

However, there is higher chance of bleeding in thread lifting than filler procedures. This is due to the characteristics of the thread lifting procedure. Not only the length of the threads is long but also the threads which inevitably pass through several blood vessels in their pathway for lifting procedure. Blood vessels get damaged from cannulas or needles but damages from thread cogs are also possible.

Among these, the most caution should be taken not to damage the superficial temporal artery/vein and the zygomatico-orbital artery.

Considering the course of the superficial temporary artery, it is inevitable that thread should cross the superficial temporal artery in the midface thread lifting (Fig. 5.1). The superficial temporal artery is rather the thick vessel; therefore, it is protruded to the subcutaneous fat (second layer) although it is enclosed by the superficial temporal fascia (third layer) (Fig. 5.2).

## 5.2 Superficial Temporal Artery

Due to the relationship among blood vessels, the fascia, and the subcutaneous fat layer, clinicians should be cautious when progressing cannulas and needles in this area.

When bleeding occurs during the process, it is important to decide whether to continue with the procedure or to pull the thread out. Depending on the location of the bleeding and blood vessel suspected to be damaged, active hemostasis or even removing the thread may be required.

In general, when inserting the cannula, the likelihood of vessel injury is relatively low as the superficial temporal artery is thick and elastic. The use of blunt cannula with pinch technique can reduce the possibility of vascular injury.

However, when a needle or a sharp cannula of needle type is used in the procedure, the possibility of vascular injury increases. If severe bleeding occurs during an anchoring procedure in the temporal area, strict hemostasis must be done; otherwise a large hematoma can occur after the

© Springer Nature Singapore Pte Ltd. 2019
B. Kim et al., *The Art and Science of Thread Lifting*, https://doi.org/10.1007/978-981-13-0614-3_5

**Fig. 5.1** Important arteries in thread lifting. The thread must cross these arteries when midface thread lifting is performed. (Published with kind permission of © Kwan- Hyun Youn 2018. All rights reserved)

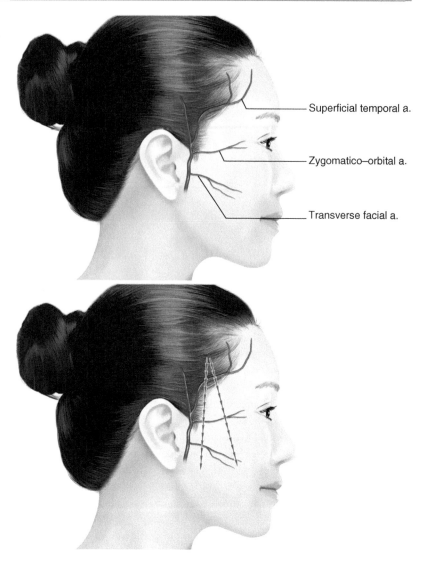

Superficial temporal a.

Zygomatico–orbital a.

Transverse facial a.

**Fig. 5.2** Depth of the superficial temporal artery. (Published with kind permission of © Kwan- Hyun Youn 2018. All rights reserved)

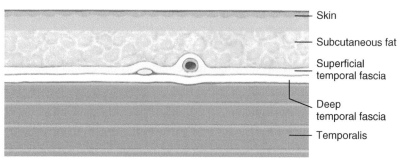

Skin

Subcutaneous fat

Superficial temporal fascia

Deep temporal fascia

Temporalis

procedure, resulting in discomfort and low satisfaction of the patients.

## 5.3 Transverse Facial Artery

Transverse facial artery is branched from the superficial temporal artery within the parotid gland and runs embedded in it. Therefore, when the thread passes over the parotid gland, it must be through the subcutaneous fat layer. If any damage occurs in the parotid gland, the transverse facial artery is also in danger, resulting in sialocele and even hematoma.

After emerging from the parotid gland, the transverse facial artery still travels beneath the SMAS and facial expression muscles. If the thread is inserted into the subcutaneous fat layer after clearly recognizing it, vascular injury can be avoided.

## 6.1 Injury to Facial Nerves

When performing midface lifting, precaution must be taken not to damage facial nerves (Fig. 6.1).

When the main temporal branch of the facial nerves is damaged, complications such as eyelid sagging and drooping eyebrows can occur (Fig. 6.2).

In case of thread lifting, the incidence rate of side effects seems to be lower than surgery. This is because thread lifting procedure is minimally invasive and facial nerve ramifies into numerous branches and anastomosis exists between them.

**Fig. 6.1** Dangerous zone. (Published with kind permission of © Kwan- Hyun Youn 2018. All rights reserved)

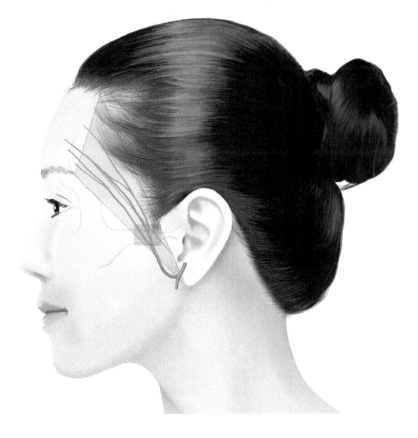

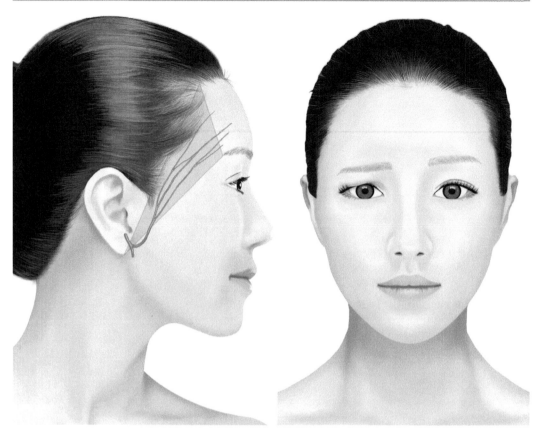

**Fig. 6.2** If temporal branches of the facial nerve are damaged in this area, the eyebrows may droop due to the weakness of the frontalis muscle. (Published with kind permission of © Kwan- Hyun Youn 2018. All rights reserved)

## 6.2    Facial Nerves in the Zygomatic Arch Area

To be able to perform thread lifting safely without nerve damages, the thread needs to be inserted through the safe facial plane. The zygomatic arch is the most likely place for nerve damage because the thickness of the soft tissues is relatively thin at this area.

When the facial nerve passes the zygomatic arch, it runs below the SMAS, and it travels very close to the bone (Figs. 6.3 and 6.4).

From the perspective of the pinch anatomy, when pinched softly, the facial nerve cannot be pulled upward from the zygomatic arch area. If progression of thread in the zygomatic arch area is made with this knowledge in mind, the possibility of nerve damage can be reduced during the procedure.

## 6.3    Technique to Reduce Nerve Injuries

When performing thread lift, we have to be cautious not to damage the facial nerve with sharp needle or careless cannula movement. It is possible to perform safe procedure by reducing the pressure on the soft tissues with pinch technique and passing threads over the zygomatic arch area carefully through gentle operation.

**Fig. 6.3** Course of the temporal branch of the facial nerve. (Published with kind permission of © Kwan-Hyun Youn 2018. All rights reserved)

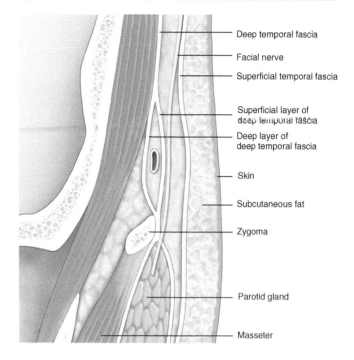

Deep temporal fascia

Facial nerve

Superficial temporal fascia

Superficial layer of deep temporal fascia

Deep layer of deep temporal fascia

Skin

Subcutaneous fat

Zygoma

Parotid gland

Masseter

**Fig. 6.4** Course of the temporal branch of the facial nerve. (Published with kind permission of © Kwan-Hyun Youn 2018. All rights reserved)

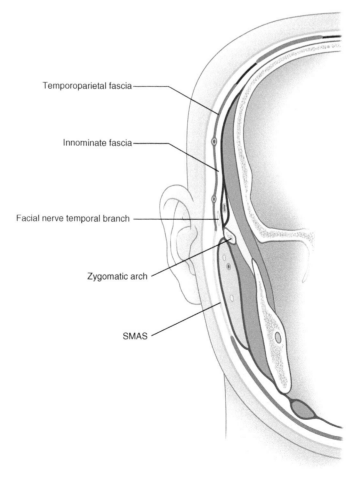

Temporoparietal fascia

Innominate fascia

Facial nerve temporal branch

Zygomatic arch

SMAS

# Part III

# Why Pinch Anatomy?

# What Is Pinch Anatomy?

The facial structures displayed in medical illustrations or revealed by cadaver dissection are their natural appearance. These are in their natural condition without exerting manipulation such as pinching or pulling on them. On the contrary, the tissue status being pulled or pinched during procedures is different from their original appearance. As well as the difference in the appearance, changes occur in the internal tissues.

In general, clinicians tend to perform aesthetic procedures while pinching the skin for the ease of the procedure. However, what happens below the skin at that time is not clearly known.

Therefore, we named the anatomy in the new status changed through pinching or pulling the tissues upward as "pinch anatomy" and studied tissue changes therefrom (Fig. 7.1).

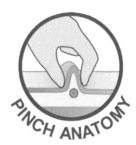

**Fig. 7.1** Logo of pinch anatomy

B. Kim et al., *The Art and Science of Thread Lifting*, https://doi.org/10.1007/978-981-13-0614-3_7

While performing thread lifting procedures, precautions must be taken against damaging the nerves and blood vessels. Especially, if the cannula containing the tread is a sharp needle type, there is higher possibility of bleeding or nerve damage.

Thread lifting is not a surgery, but a minimally invasive procedure. The advantages of minimally invasive procedures are low occurrence of complications, fast recovery, and the short procedure time. Therefore, maximizing the value of the thread lifting would be to minimize the possibility of bleeding and nerve damage.

The knowledge of the depth of major nerves and blood vessels based on facial anatomy is a prerequisite for thread lifting. In addition to this, we think that knowledge about the pinch anatomy will make the procedure to be safer and more effective. We expect that additional studies will be carried out on pinch anatomy in the future.

In summary, clinicians generally tend to pinch or pull the tissues for the ease of procedure. In such case, anatomical structure changes occur. If thread lifting is carried out in the safe layer with clear knowledge of the anatomical changes in the pinched status, damages to the blood vessels and nerves can be avoided.

Considering the depth and course of main blood vessels and nerves, in manipulating a pinch, which layer of face is pulled upward and whether blood vessels and nerves are pulled upward are very important. If they are assumed to be pulled, passing the thread in deeper layer would be safer, and if they are not pulled, inserting the thread superficially would be safer.

## 9.1 Study Method

After marking the hairline from fresh cadaver which has been frozen or fixed and shaving the hair, several points were marked at important sites for thread lifting procedure (Fig. 9.1).

After performing a gentle pinch in each area, the pulled up skin was cut at the bottom with scissors (Fig. 9.2).

While the tissue is being pulled, the skin is thought to be cut at a slightly deeper than the layer where the cannula is inserted. The exposed area was observed with the naked eye, and at the

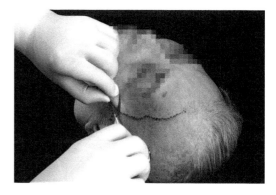

**Fig. 9.2** The method of gentle pinch and cutting of pulled up skin. (Published with kind permission of © Wonsug Jung 2018. All rights reserved)

border of the cut area, tissue specimens were collected to be examined microscopically to determine which layer of face was pulled up and cut.

## 9.2 Result

In the temple area inside the hairline, the subcutaneous fat layer was cleanly removed, and the superficial temporal artery and the superficial temporal fascia enclosing it were not damaged.

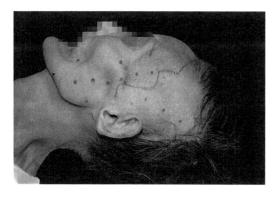

**Fig. 9.1** Sites where pinch and cut were performed. (Published with kind permission of © Wonsug Jung 2018. All rights reserved)

© Springer Nature Singapore Pte Ltd. 2019
B. Kim et al., *The Art and Science of Thread Lifting*, https://doi.org/10.1007/978-981-13-0614-3_9

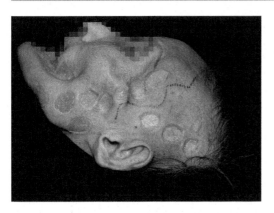

In all other areas, some amount of subcutaneous fat was not removed, and facial expression muscles were observed to be intact where muscles could be seen through barely remaining subcutaneous fat (Fig. 9.3).

**Fig. 9.3** Result of pinch and cut. (Published with kind permission of © Wonsug Jung 2018. All rights reserved)

## 10.1 Pinch Anatomy: Temple Area Inside the Hairline

While performing long thread lifting, how deep anchoring will be done is very important. This is because the temporal fascia creates much stronger fixing point than the subcutaneous fat layer. At the time of pinch, it is necessary to know which fascia in the temporal area is being pulled. The anchoring itself is a blind procedure; therefore the layer that thread hangs cannot be confirmed visually.

During performing anchoring in the temporal fascia area, there must be no damage to the superficial temporal artery which is enclosed in the superficial temporal fascia. Finding out how blood vessels and fascia move around these areas when performing a pinch helps to reduce injury of blood vessels (Figs. 10.1 and 10.2).

**Gross Finding** Temple areas inside the hairline

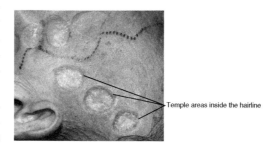

Temple areas inside the hairline

**Fig. 10.1** Location of the superficial temporal artery in the temporal area. (Published with kind permission of © Kwan- Hyun Youn 2018. All rights reserved)

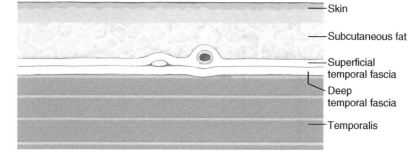

Skin

Subcutaneous fat

Superficial temporal fascia

Deep temporal fascia

Temporalis

**Fig. 10.2**
Recommended area for
anchoring. Anchoring is
done between the frontal
and parietal branches of
the superficial temporal
artery. (Published with
kind permission of ©
Kwan- Hyun Youn 2018.
All rights reserved)

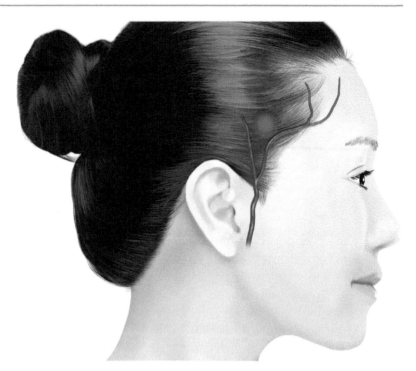

- Through cutting after pinching, the subcutaneous fat layer was removed, and the superficial
  temporal fascia was exposed. Damage to the
  superficial temporal fascia was not visible.
- Only the subcutaneous fat layer was presumed
  to be pulled upward by the pinch.
- This shows that the superficial temporal fascia
  was not pulled upward easily by a gentle pinch.
- Based on the lack of difference in the border
  of cut skin and the subcutaneous fat layer, it
  can be assumed that the pinch separated the
  subcutaneous fat layer from the fascia beneath.
- The superficial temporal artery is surrounded
  by the superficial temporal fascia, but it
  sticks out to the subcutaneous fat layer. The
  entire fat layer was removed without damage
  to the artery, which supports that the pinch
  caused separation of the subcutaneous fat
  layer and the superficial temporal fascia.

**Histologic Finding**  The temple area inside the
hairline

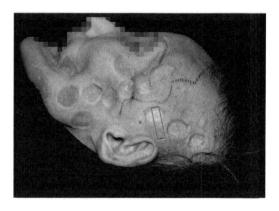

- The red square indicates the orientation of the
  tissue specimen.
- There is almost no subcutaneous fat layer in
  the temple area inside the hairline.
- The superficial temporal fascia (STF) splits to
  surround the superficial temporal artery
  (STA), and it is not damaged from cutting
  after pinching.
- The temporal branches (black arrows) of the
  facial nerve travel in between the STF and the
  deep temporal fascia (DTF).

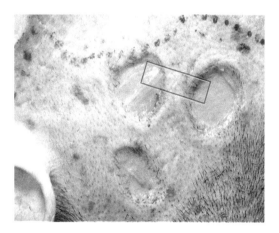

- In another cadaver, the skin was pinched deeply and cut at one point to determine whether there is difference in movement of tissue layers according to the strength of pinch method (Fig. 10.3).
- When the cutting was done after gentle pinching using the ordinary method, only the subcutaneous fat layer was cut, and there was no damage to the STF and the STA. When the pinch was manipulated deeply, however, the STF was cut, and the deep temporal fascia (DTF) was exposed. The exposed deep temporal fascia (DTF) was not damaged at all.
- Depending on the strength of the pinch method, the pulled up layer can be different.

**Fig. 10.3** The temporal area where two different pinch methods were applied. On the left side, the skin was pinched gently; on the right side, the skin was pinched deeply. (Published with kind permission of © Wonsug Jung 2018. All rights reserved)

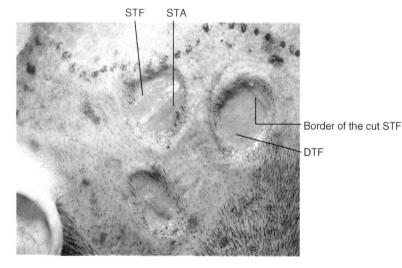

- The red square indicates the orientation of the tissue specimen.
- The left side of the tissue specimen is the area where a gentle pinch was performed, and the right side is where a deep pinch was applied.

- Only the subcutaneous fat layer was cut, and there was no damage to the STA and STF in the left, but it can be seen that the STF was removed, and the DTF was exposed in the right.
- Thin temporoparietalis muscle was observed in the same layer as the STF.

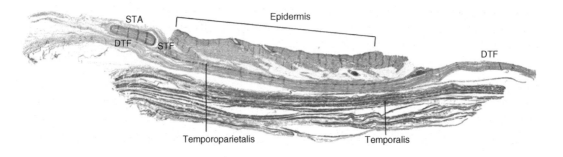

## 10.2    Pinch Anatomy: Temple Area

- This is an area which is bounded by the orbital rim, the zygomatic arch, and the hairline.
- Important anatomical structures such as the temporal branch of the facial nerve and the frontal branch of the superficial temporal artery traverse this area.
- The temporal branches of the facial nerve pass deep to the superficial temporal fascia, and when the skin was cut after being pinched, there was no damage to the superficial temporal fascia.

**Gross Finding**  Temple area

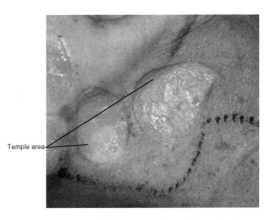

- In the area where the subcutaneous fat exists to a certain extent, only part of the subcutaneous fat layer is removed together with the skin when pinched and cut.
- Part of the subcutaneous fat layer remains, and there is no damage to the superficial temporal fascia which is located deep to it.
- Therefore, the superficial temporal artery which is enclosed in the superficial temporal fascia and the temporal branch of the facial nerve which travels deep to the STF are not damaged.

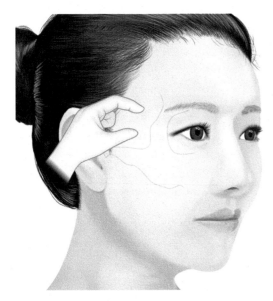

## 10.3   Pinch Anatomy: Zygomatic Arch Area

Due to the possibility of injury to the facial nerve, the tissue change from pinch in this area raises the most curiosity. As the temporal branch of the facial nerve runs beneath the superficial temporal fascia in this area, whether the superficial temporal fascia is pulled is important. Especially, as it is before the temporal branch of the facial nerve makes many branches, a nerve damage in this area can potentially cause a relatively serious complication.

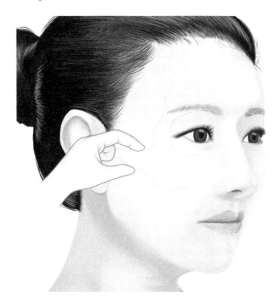

- As it can be seen in Fig. 10.4, the facial nerve crosses the zygomatic arch and traverses the innominate fascia to reach just beneath the SMAS in the temporal area.
- When thread lifting is performed using the temporal anchoring method, the cannula proceeds toward the lower cheek after passing the zygomatic arch. The facial nerve crosses the zygomatic arch deep to the SMAS and superficial temporal fascia. Therefore, when the cannula proceeds within the subcutaneous layer after separating the subcutaneous fat layer from the SMAS through pinching, there is less chance to cause injury to the facial nerve.

**Gross Finding**   Zygomatic arch area

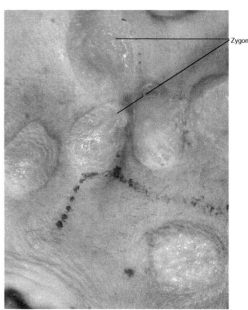

Zygoma

- In the area where the subcutaneous fat layer exists to a certain extent, only some of the subcutaneous fat layer is removed together with the skin when cutting is performed after pinching.
- Some remaining subcutaneous fat is observed with the naked eye, and the SMAS which is located more deeply is not damaged.
- Accordingly, the temporal branch of the facial nerve which travels deep to the SMAS is not damaged.
- Muscles are seen through the area where large amount of the subcutaneous fat layer is removed.

**Histologic Finding**   Zygomatic arch area

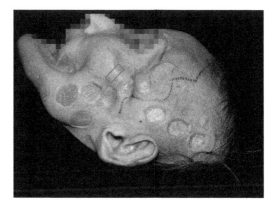

**Fig. 10.4** Course of the temporal branch of the facial nerve. (Published with kind permission of © Kwan- Hyun Youn 2018. All rights reserved)

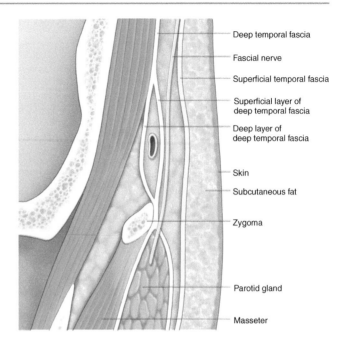

Deep temporal fascia

Fascial nerve

Superficial temporal fascia

Superficial layer of deep temporal fascia

Deep layer of deep temporal fascia

Skin

Subcutaneous fat

Zygoma

Parotid gland

Masseter

- The red square indicates the orientation of the tissue specimen.
- After pinching, some of the subcutaneous fat layer is removed through cutting.

- In the area where the muscles are seen through thin subcutaneous fat, there is no damage to the muscle.
- The temporal branch of the facial nerve travels deep to the SMAS.

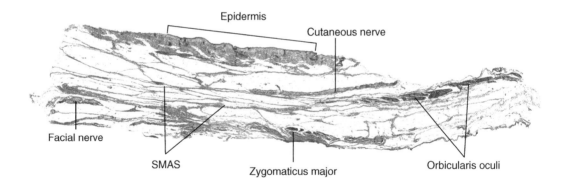

Epidermis

Cutaneous nerve

Facial nerve

SMAS

Zygomaticus major

Orbicularis oculi

## 10.4 Pinch Anatomy: Sub-zygomatic Arch Area

The sub-zygomatic arch area is usually depressed creating a sunken cheek. This is an area with relatively severe adhesion due to abundant fibrotic tissues. Therefore, when cog threads are hung in this area, it can tolerate pulling force fairly well, and a good lifting outcome can be expected.

On the other hand, if the process of the thread lifting is carried out without clear knowledge of the characteristics of this area, side effects such as sinking can easily occur for the same reason. Therefore, an optimal procedure must be performed based on various skills such as the pinch manipulation and design know-how.

- Therefore, the parotid gland which is located deep to the SMAS is not damaged.

## 10.5   Pinch Anatomy: Cheek Area

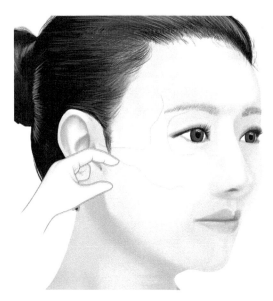

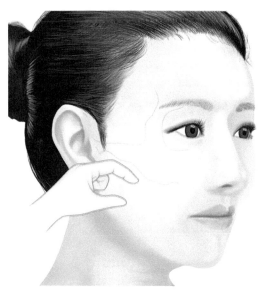

**Gross Finding** Sub-zygomatic arch

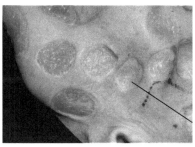

Sub-zygomatic arch

- In the right top side of the cut surface, the dermis and subcutaneous fat tissues are cut obliquely. This is the result of this area not being pulled upward as much as the other areas at the time of pinching due to the dense fibrotic tissues.
- In the area where the subcutaneous fat layer exists to a certain extent, only some of the subcutaneous fat layer is removed together with the skin when cutting is performed after pinching.
- Some remaining subcutaneous fat is observed with the naked eye, and the SMAS which is located more deeply is not damaged.

For the cheek area, it is advisable to keep in mind the location and the depth of the masseter muscle and the parotid gland.

As illustrated in Fig. 4.5, the parotid duct, the facial nerve branches, etc. travel embedded in the parotid gland; therefore inserting and proceeding thread through the subcutaneous layer can be safe.

When this area is pinched, it can be seen that only the subcutaneous fat layer is pulled, but in case of those patients with thin subcutaneous fat layer, the depth for the procedure needs careful adjustment to suit the individual. It is advised to proceed the thread with sense of penetration through the tissue area which is lifted after gentle pinching.

In this area, caution must be exercised not to damage the parotid glands, the parotid duct, the facial nerve, the transverse facial artery, etc. The above structures travel inside the parotid gland, and after they emerge from the gland, they run covered by the SMAS

The layers pulled up with pinch manipulation must be kept in mind, and a thread should be inserted into the proper plane during the thread lift procedure.

**Histologic Finding** Cheek

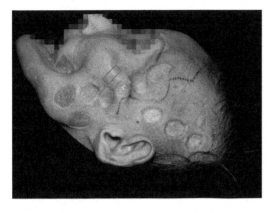

- The red square indicates the orientation of the tissue specimen.

- In the bottom of the cutout surface, the dermis and subcutaneous fat tissues are cut obliquely. This is the result of this area not being pulled upward as much as other areas at the time of pinching due to the dense fibrotic tissues.
- In the area where the subcutaneous fat layer exists to a certain extent, only some of the subcutaneous fat layer is removed together with the skin when pinched and cut.
- Some remaining subcutaneous fat is observed with the naked eye, and the SMAS which is located more deeply is not damaged.
- Both the SMAS and the parotidomasseteric fascia are thick over the parotid gland, but they become thin over the masseter.
- The buccal branches of the facial nerve which travel with the parotid duct can be observed.

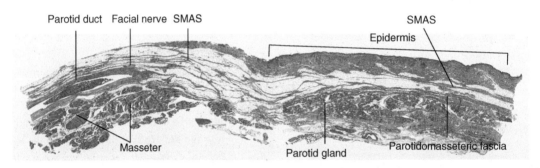

## 10.6 Pinch Anatomy: Lower Cheek Area

In this area, caution must be taken not to damage the buccal and marginal mandibular branches of the facial nerve. The branches of the facial nerve travel inside the parotid gland, and after they come out of the gland, they run beneath the SMAS.

The layers pulled up with pinch manipulation must be kept in mind, and a thread should be inserted into proper plane during the thread lift procedure

**Gross Finding**

- In the area where the subcutaneous fat layer exists to a certain extent, only some of the subcutaneous fat layer is removed together with the skin when cutting is performed after pinching.
- Some remaining subcutaneous fat is observed with the naked eye, and the SMAS which is located more deeply is not damaged.

- Therefore, the buccal and marginal mandibular branch of the facial nerve which travel deep to the SMAS is not damaged.

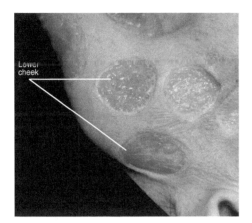

# Pinch Anatomy Summary

## 11.1 Areas Where Pinch Anatomy Is Important

Pinch anatomy is meaningful in that it can assist with safe procedures. Especially, it helps to prevent blood vessel damage in the temporal area and nerve damage in the zygomatic arch area. It is related to the movement of blood vessels and nerves in the facial layer when pinch is applied to those areas.

### 11.1.1 Temple Area Inside the Hairline

Pinch anatomy in the temporal area shows various key facts. The result of cutting after pinching is shown in Fig. 10.3. Note that fat around the superficial temporal artery is removed almost completely. In other words, the fat layer located at the same depth as the blood vessel is damaged, while the blood vessel itself is intact (Figs. 11.1, 11.2, and 11.3).

When deep pinch was applied to the temporal area, interesting result was observed. The superficial temporal fascia was also removed along with the skin and subcutaneous fat (Fig. 11.4).

Figure 11.4 provides a lot of information. Although the method of fixing a thread in the fascia in the temporal area is the most effective, it is not technically easy. Also, as it is a blind technique, when anchoring is done, whether the thread actually hangs in the superficial temporal fascia or the thread reaches up to the deep temporal fascia cannot be directly confirmed visually. It is clear that the thread must be hung in the fascia to make a harder fixing point. However, whether the thread is actually hung in the fascia is difficult to know even during the procedure.

Based on the overall pinch anatomy findings in the temporal area, the following conclusions can be drawn.

1. When a pinch is done, a certain area of the temporal tissue loosens and this area is pulled up.
   - When the pinch is gently applied, the interface between the subcutaneous fat and the superficial temporal fascia becomes loose, and the gap is created between them.
   - When the pinch is deeply applied, the superficial temporal fascia is separated from the deep temporal fascia.
2. When the gentle pinch is applied, the superficial temporal vessel encased by the superficial temporal fascia remains at the bottom, while subcutaneous fat is pulled upward with the skin.
3. With the knowledge of pulled up layers with different pinch methods, clinicians can be confident in targeting the temporal fascia for anchoring a thread.

B. Kim et al., *The Art and Science of Thread Lifting*, https://doi.org/10.1007/978-981-13-0614-3_11

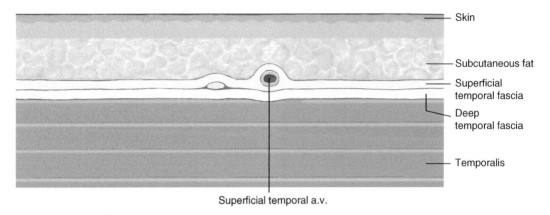

Superficial temporal a.v.

**Fig. 11.1** Location of the superficial temporal artery in the temporal area. (Published with kind permission of © Kwan-Hyun Youn 2018. All rights reserved)

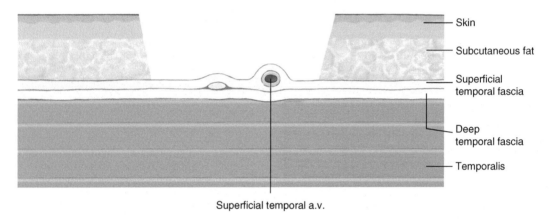

Superficial temporal a.v.

**Fig. 11.2** The result of cutting after pinching. (Published with kind permission of © Kwan- Hyun Youn 2018. All rights reserved)

## 11.1.2  Zygomatic Arch Area

The facial nerve passes across the zygomatic arch. When a surgical facial lifting is performed, the facial nerve can be injured causing frontalis muscle weakness and eyebrows sagging.

Also in case of performing absorbable thread lifting, caution must be taken when the cannula is crossing the zygomatic arch. The facial nerve runs beneath the superficial temporal fascia, and it does not get lifted with gentle pinching (Fig. 11.5). Therefore, the cannula can cross the zygomatic arch without damaging the facial nerve if it is advanced in the subcutaneous fat layer.

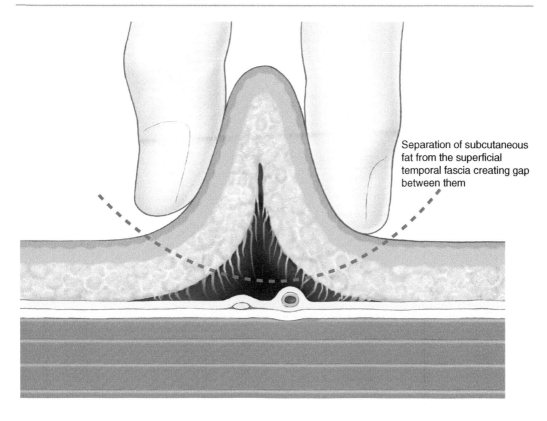

Separation of subcutaneous fat from the superficial temporal fascia creating gap between them

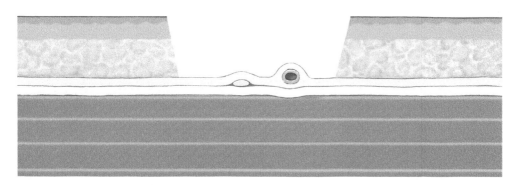

**Fig. 11.3** The proposed mechanism of intact superficial temporal artery with surrounding fat completely removed. (Published with kind permission of © Kwan- Hyun Youn 2018. All rights reserved)

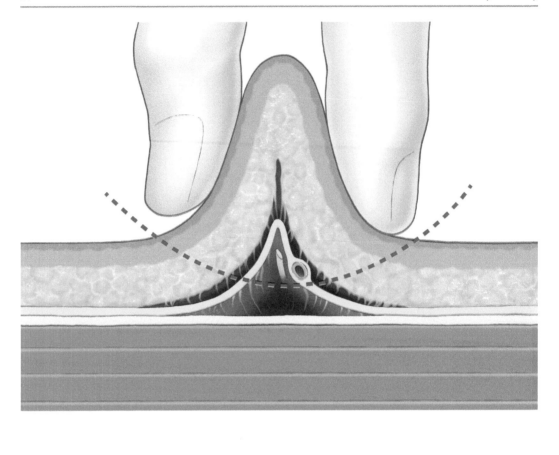

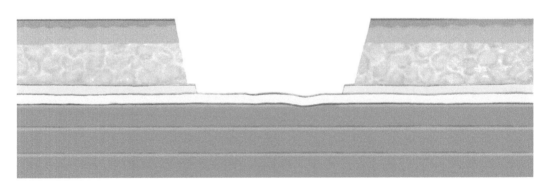

**Fig. 11.4** The proposed mechanism of removal of the superficial temporal fascia. (Published with kind permission of © Kwan- Hyun Youn 2018. All rights reserved)

**Fig. 11.5** Pinch on the zygomatic arch area (Published with kind permission of © Kwan- Hyun Youn 2018. All rights reserved)

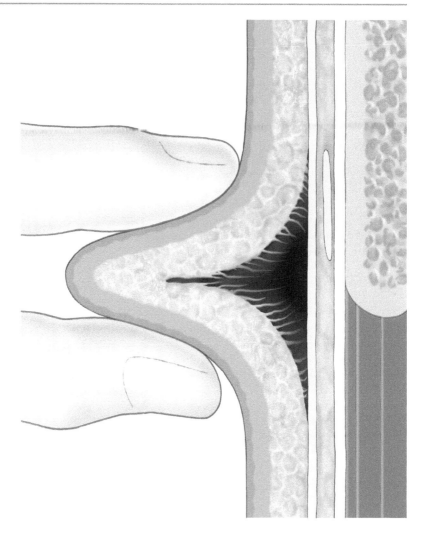

**Summary**

Area where manipulation of pinching is useful

- Temple area inside the hairline
  - Pinching may reduce the likelihood of damaging the superficial temporal vessel when making a puncture and anchoring a thread.

- Pinching may help the thread to proceed at an appropriate depth without damaging blood vessels.
- Zygomatic arch area
  - When gentle pinch is applied, the facial nerve located deep to the SMAS is not pulled upward.
  - Pinching may reduce the possibility of facial nerve injury.

# Part IV

# Understanding Absorbable Threads

## 12.1 Trend of Thread Lifting

| | First-generation lifting thread | Second-generation lifting thread | Third-generation lifting thread | Fourth-generation lifting thread |
|---|---|---|---|---|
| Shape | | | | |
| Feature | Thin mono-thread | Thread in a twister shape | Cutting thread with cog | Bi-directional molding cog |
| Key effects | Improve fine wrinkles | Skin regeneration | Lifting | Lifting |
| | Skin elasticity | Skin elasticity | Improve fine wrinkles | Improve deep wrinkles |
| | | | V-line | V-line |
| | | | Skin regeneration | Skin regeneration |
| | | | Skin elasticity | Skin elasticity |

The present day can be called the golden days of the PDO threads. As there are various types and product groups, even selecting is not easy. Therefore, to select the adequate PDO lifting products, clear understanding of the characteristics of various threads is required. Threads can be classified by several standards, and threads can be selected based on the purpose of the procedure.

Standards for classifying the PDO threads are in Table 12.1.

### 12.1.1 Distinction of Threads

The top picture in Fig. 12.1 means mono-thread. By inserting into the subcutaneous or SMAS layer and causing tissue reactions, lifting or tightening effects can be obtained.

The bottom picture in Fig. 12.1 is a cog thread. A cog which looks like a thorn is produced by a cutting or molding method in accordance with the direction to pull. If it is pulled after inserting the thread in the facial tissue, tissues will be hanged to the threads due to the function of cogs.

The top picture in Fig. 12.2 shows a unidirectional cog thread in which the direction of the cogs is consistent from the beginning to the end. This was largely used in the initial cog thread lifting procedures. The function of making a fixing point was weak, and there was insufficient explanation about mechanisms. This is not used much currently.

© Springer Nature Singapore Pte Ltd. 2019
B. Kim et al., *The Art and Science of Thread Lifting*, https://doi.org/10.1007/978-981-13-0614-3_12

**Table 12.1** Classification of absorbable threads

| Classifying standards | | |
|---|---|---|
| 1. Existence of cog | Mono-thread | Cog thread |
| 2. Direction of cog | Uni-directional cog thread | Bi-directional cog thread |
| 3. Diversity of cog directions | Zigzag type cog thread | Bi-directional cog thread |
| 4. Twisting of thread | Simple type | Twister type |
| 5. Manufacturing method of cog | Cutting method | Molding method |
| 6. Length | Long thread for anchoring | Short thread |
| 7. Shape of needle | Cannula type | Needle type |
| 8. Ingredient and duration | PDO | PLLA |

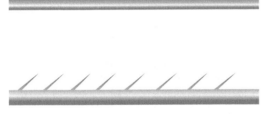

**Fig. 12.1**  Mono-thread and cog thread

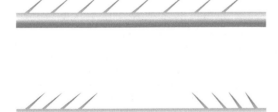

**Fig. 12.2**  Uni-directional cog thread vs bi-directional cog thread

The bottom figure in Fig. 12.2 shows a bi-directional cog thread. This product is used mostly in cog thread lifting. Cogs in different directions are made on one thread, and they have a function of gathering tissues to the middle area of the bi-directional cogs.

Figure 12.3 shows various bi-directional cogs.

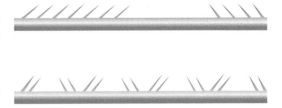

**Fig. 12.3**  Bi-directional cog thread and zigzag type thread

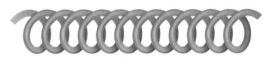

**Fig. 12.4**  Simple type (mono-thread) and twister type

The top picture is the ordinary bi-directional cogs. The bottom picture is in the similar form to the bi-directional cogs but is made in the form of continuously changing directions. It is often called a zigzag type thread. Rather than serving the lifting function of pulling tissues, it is largely used for the purpose of fixing the lifting effect made by bi-directional cog threads and preventing sinking of the skin.

The top picture in Fig. 12.4 shows a mono-thread.

The bottom picture shows a PDO thread in a twisted form. Products with various names exist. With internal structure of twisting type, it is expected to form collagen better, and it has a slight volumizing effect. Therefore, by inserting many of them in one area simultaneously, it sometimes has an effect which is similar to fillers, and it sometimes shows effect of pressing the sagged cheek area by using the feature that is harder than ordinary mono-threads. It is produced to be thicker and harder than ordinary PDO threads.

The top picture in Fig. 12.5 shows cutting type thread among production forms of cogs. As the cogs are labile, when they are inserted into tissues and pulled, they hang on tissues well. On the other hand, as the thickness of the thread body is

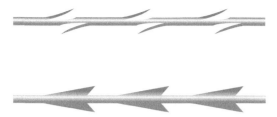

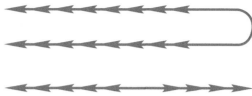

**Fig. 12.6** Long thread and short thread

**Fig. 12.5** Cutting thread and molding thread

becoming thin due to cutting, tensile strength is reduced.

The bottom figure is a molding thread which has been positioned to be a key thread among cog threads. It is manufactured in the method of molding while simultaneously pressing the body and cogs of the thread. It shows better effects than the cutting thread in terms of tensile strength and retentivity.

The top picture in Fig. 12.6 is a PDO bi-directional cog thread called a long thread. However, it does not use the functions of the bi-directional cogs and actually uses the functions of unidirectional cogs by fixing the area without cog in the middle of the thread to the fascia in the temporal area. This is a thread used in fixed type lifting.

The bottom picture is a PDO bi-directional cog threads ordinarily referred as short threads. Using the mechanisms of the bi-directional cogs, lifting effects are created by causing the tissues to gather at the middle area of the thread.

The top picture in Fig. 12.7 shows a sharp needle type cog contained in a cannula. As it is a needle type, it easily passes tissues during procedures. However, the chance of bleeding is relatively high compared to the thread contained in a cannula.

The bottom picture shows a cog thread contained in a blunt cannula. This is harder for passing tissues during procedures, but it has advantage of causing less bleeding.

### 12.1.2 Current Trend

Based on the current trend of absorbable threads, cog threads are used mainly. Mono-threads are

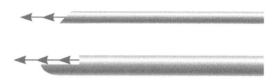

**Fig. 12.7** Needle type thread and cannula type thread

still advertised as being used for lifting purpose; based on the prior use, it is thought to be more accurate to say that it is used for the purpose of tightening to contract inner tissues.

For strong and sustained lifting effects, a molding type PDO thread which is stronger and longer lasting is developed and used. Based on such development from technical and material engineering perspectives, various indications and procedure methods are being made. For example, recently, absorbable threads are being used for other purposes, not simply lifting but reducing the nostrils and raising the nose, etc. For such contents used in advertisements, our clinicians should have attitudes of attempting to study and verify the effects of the new techniques and durations.

On one hand, ingredients which can last longer are being paid attention as materials for absorbable thread lifting. As the existing fillers or medical devices, materials which are verified for safety are largely used. Cosmetic medicine in Korea is developing at a rapid rate. This is not an outcome achieved not only by medical practitioners.

This is an outcome achieved through convergence of complicated intermix of power of engineers who plan and develop products and marketing-related people who commercialize them, etc.

## 13.1 Physical Characteristics of PDO

The thread of PDO ingredient has been used as a suture for a long period and it is proved to be safe. It lasts longer compared to Dexon and Vicryl and completely absorbs after 6 months and disappears from the body. Therefore, it has been used for closing the area which requires long tension.

Moreover, as PDO threads can be manufactured in a surface which is soft and monofilament in form, the risk of latent infection which can occur by settling of germs on the surface of the thread is low. Accordingly, it has been accepted for its safety and sustainability as a suture.

## 13.2 Functions of PDO

In general, a PDO is known to cause changes to the dermis. As discovered in several studies, it has effects of improving pores or fine wrinkles.

Especially, it is known to increase thickness of the papillary dermis, which is done through the method of fostering collagen formation in the dermal matrix.

## 13.3 Tissue Changes After Inserting PDO Threads

In the journal, the authors explain tissue changes after inserting the PDO thread into the subcutaneous layer.

This is an excellent study which can explain the changes to the skin and the subcutaneous layer after submitting the PDO thread. Based on this, significant portion of thread lifting mechanisms could be explained.

The changes after inserting the PDO can be summarized as follows.

## 13.4 Histologic Findings After PDO Thread Insertion

1. Many PMN cells, including eosinophile, are gathered making granulation tissues around the thread which is inserted. In the granulation tissues, newly made collagenous connective tissues are abundantly observed.

© Springer Nature Singapore Pte Ltd. 2019
B. Kim et al., *The Art and Science of Thread Lifting*, https://doi.org/10.1007/978-981-13-0614-3_13

2. The newly made collagenous connective tissues converge into the pre-existing fibrous connective tissues nearby (merging effect). Through merging effect, an inflammatory reaction is in progress to the surrounding area where the thread is inserted, and mechanotransduction (=cell signal delivery happens when granulation tissues are formed) starts and spreads as waves to surrounding tissues.

3. Inside the granulation tissues which are newly made near the inserted thread, fibroblasts and myofibroblasts show. Myofibroblast is mostly clearly related to a wound contracture in the wound healing process, and it is a cell which serves a key role of causing elasticity in the area of the procedure and tight skin after the skin regeneration procedure.

4. The cross-sectional area size of capillaries is larger in experimental group where the PDO thread was inserted than control group. Also, many eosinophils were observed which shows effects for inducing fibrosis in the wound healing process.

5. There was fat cell denaturation by granulation tissue only in the area where the thread was inserted, and there was no change to fat cells away from granulation tissues (Fig. 13.1, Table 13.1).

**Table 13.1** Summary of histologic changes after inserting PDO

| Newly developed fibrous connective tissue |
|---|
| Merging with existing fibrous connective tissue |
| Tissue contraction by myofibroblast |
| Increased capillary vessel size |
| Fat cell denaturation |

**Fig. 13.1** Schematic diagram of change after mono-thread insertion. (Five tissue changes mentioned above are shown)

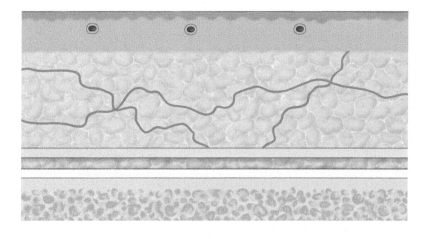

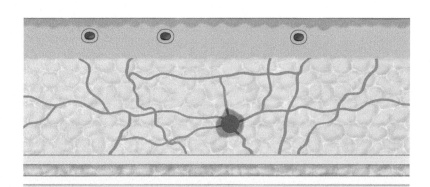

## 14.1 PLLA as a Suture Material

Once it is discovered that volume loss is the most crucial element of aging, various materials were used to create volume in the face.

PLLA (poly-L-lactic acid: Sculptra®) is used as a material for volumizing. PLLA can be biodegraded and it is an adequate material for the living body. In general, after being inserted into the body, it forms collagen, and it is known to be sustained for 2 years. After being inserted into the body, PLLA forms type 1 collagen and type 3 collagen, and it is known to cause almost no or very small amount of inflammatory reaction to the surrounding tissues.

Kulkarni and colleagues also have stated that when PLLA was injected into the subcutaneous tissue, there is a very weak inflammatory response initially, but it disappears as time goes on. Gogolewski et al. also observed changes after injecting PLLA. It was stated that as PLLA was decomposed, collagen settlement increased but that no acute inflammatory response was observed.

Hyaluronic acid ingredient can also make some collagen around the injected area, but this differs from what is made by the PLLA ingredient. Volume formation using a hyaluronic acid filler is mostly by the hyaluronic acid itself and partially by newly formed collagen. On the other hand, PLLA ingredients differ in that they are decomposed slowly over a period of 2 years and collagens mostly fill the space.

© Springer Nature Singapore Pte Ltd. 2019
B. Kim et al., *The Art and Science of Thread Lifting*, https://doi.org/10.1007/978-981-13-0614-3_14

# Type of Absorbable Thread Products

## 15.1 QT Lift (= VOV Lift, = BLUE ROSE® FORTE)

### 15.1.1 Features

QT lift or QTL (=VOV lift, = BLUE ROSE® FORTE) is a molding type PDO thread. In this product, the sustained duration and tensile strength, which were weak features in the existing cutting type threads, are significantly improving. Through a pressure molding method, while constantly maintaining the thickness of the body of the thread, cogs are strong and durable (Fig. 15.1). As cogs are many in number and close together, they hang the tissues evenly in many areas.

Through in vitro study, it was discovered that it has stronger tensile strength (Fig. 15.2) and longer duration than cutting type cog threads (Table 15.1).

A long thread to fix the temporal fascia and a short thread for simple insertion and tying, etc. are commercialized (Table 15.2).

### 15.1.2 Advantages Determined by the Authors

There are several problems with absorbable thread lifting.

① Insufficient effect
② Short duration
③ Side effects such as dimpling
④ Bruising and swelling

Among these, molding type thread achieved improvement from perspectives of effects and duration. As seen Fig. 15.2, not only the tensile strength is five times the existing cutting

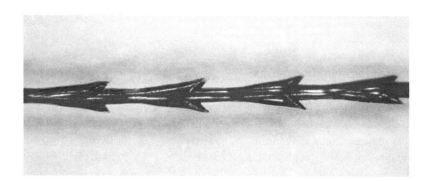

**Fig. 15.1** QT lift = VOV lift = BLUE ROSE® FORTE. (Close shot. A strong thread body and a cog shape made by pressure molding method can be seen)

© Springer Nature Singapore Pte Ltd. 2019
B. Kim et al., *The Art and Science of Thread Lifting*, https://doi.org/10.1007/978-981-13-0614-3_15

**Fig. 15.2** Tensile
strength. Ref. R&D
dept. of Feel tech Co.,
Ltd., 2015. (Source:
2015 research materials
of Blue Rose Porte
manufacturer)

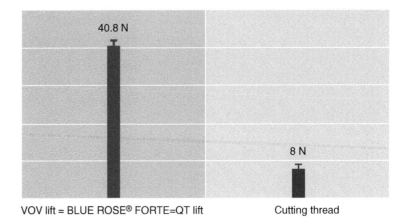

VOV lift = BLUE ROSE® FORTE=QT lift                          Cutting thread

**Table 15.1**  Long lasting

|          | Initial shape | After 30 days | After 90 days |
|----------|---------------|---------------|---------------|
| VOV lift | 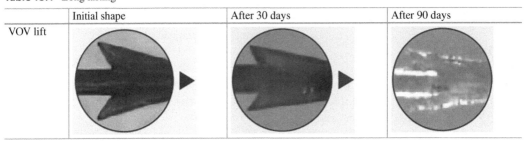 | | |

Long-lasting, durable sculpted cogs
VOV lift stays in perfect shape and improving its duration
Source: Esthetics Co., Ltd.

**Table 15.2**  Characteristics of QT lift = VOV lift = BLUE ROSE® FORTE

| Thread and Cannula | |
|---|---|
| Characteristics of QT lift = VOV lift = BLUE ROSE® FORTE [18G/19G] | |
| Characteristics of QT lift = VOV lift = BLUE ROSE® FORTE [410 mm] | |

Source: 2015 research materials of Blue Rose Porte manufacturer

type thread, but also the duration of cog is relatively long.

In case of QT lift (=VOV lift, = BLUE ROSE® FORTE), which is a PDO thread in pressure molding method, the important advantages are that it is strong and has a long duration. And it is relatively thin compared to other threads which have the same strength. Therefore, it is possible to do the procedure using a smaller cannula. Also, as the cog is strong, a procedure using the tying method mentioned later is possible. When performing a procedure using a short thread, as a way to strengthen the function of the fixing point, the tying method is often used. Both the complex skill in the form of fixing at the deep temporal fascia using a long thread and a skill of simply inserting into fat and pulling can be used. Namely, this is a thread which is useful for both beginners and experienced practitioners.

**http://sthepharm.com**

## 15.2   Silhouette Soft®

### 15.2.1   Features

Silhouette Soft® is made of PLLA ingredients. It is the same ingredient as a collagen stimulator which was sold under the name Sculptra® in the past, and it has a longer duration than the PDO.

It has cogs in unique form which is different from ordinary cogs (Fig. 15.3). These cogs are called cones and are not fixed in their positions. Each cone drives freely between knots in the middle of the thread, As 12 cm needle is attached in both ends, procedures can be done without the help of supplementary cannulas or needles. Rather than a true lifting, it brings lifting effects by gathering tissues based on the soft tissue repositioning concept (Fig. 15.4).

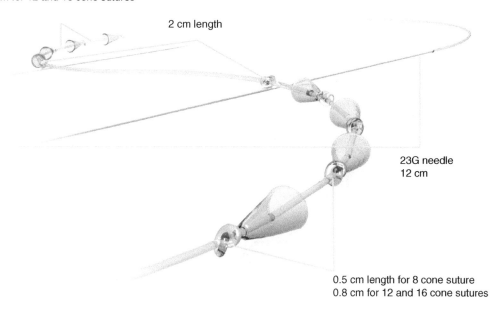

**Fig. 15.3**   Exterior and structure of Silhouette Soft®. (Source: Silhouette Soft® /SINCLAIR)

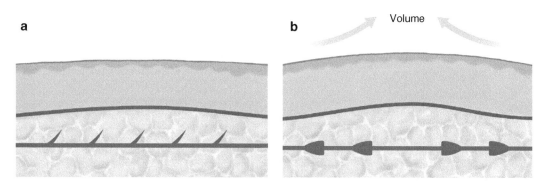

**Fig. 15.4**   Mechanisms of Silhouette Soft®. (**a**) It is a method of pulling after inserting the cog thread. (**b**) Silhouette Soft® procedure is a method of repositioning by pulling tissues at both sides)

From a perspective of materials, PLLA threads are harder than PDO threads. Also, due to lower elasticity, if PLLA are bended or pulled hard, the risk of being broken is higher than the PDO. On the contrary, duration is longer than the PDO threads. It is well known for the function of collagen formation through stimulating surrounding tissues.

### 15.2.2 Advantages Determined by the Authors

The biggest advantage is that the procedures using the Silhouette Soft® are simple and allow diverse designs. As needles are attached at the both ends of the thread, procedures can be done simply without additional devices. Since the ends are sharp, there is no problem with proceeding through the subcutaneous layer. When the procedure is performed adequately, there is less pain and bleeding due to the needle size is fine.

It is more suitable for patients that require tissue repositioning rather than lifting procedures with fixing points. For example, it is useful for treatments like gathering under eye tissues and pulling sagged lower cheeks upward by pushing upward. Complicated designs which are difficult to achieve with other types of threads can be achieved more easily by using Silhouette Soft®. This is due to the advantage of the soft and flexible needles come with the Silhouette Soft® which makes it relatively easy to proceed in curved areas.

Also, it is advantageous for procedures such as nose tip reshaping procedure, sagged neck lifting, etc. Apart from the above pros, as it is a needle type,

it should be noted that severe bleeding can occur during procedure if the adjustment of depth fails.

**https://www.sinclairpharma.com/silhouette-soft**

## 15.3  N-Cog Lift

### 15.3.1 Features

This is the first-generation PDO threads in the country. It is manufactured by cutting method. It has various product groups, and there are many areas in which procedures can be performed. It can also be used for lifting sensitive areas which are difficult to do with other threads such as periorbital area.

Bi-directional cogs and zigzag type cogs are widely used (Figs. 15.5 and 15.6), and procedures are simple.

### 15.3.2 Advantages Determined by the Authors

The procedure is simple and convenient. N-cog threads have a versatile range of products designed to treat different area of concerns. Various techniques are systematically established; it is suitable for those who just start cog threads procedure.

Although the holding power of cutting cog threads is relatively weaker than that of molding cog threads, a good result can be obtained by using suitable techniques and a sufficient volume of threads.

**http://www.nfinders.com/eng**

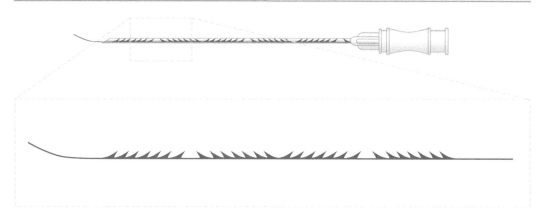

**Fig. 15.5**  N-cog lift. (Source: N-Finders Co, Ltd.)

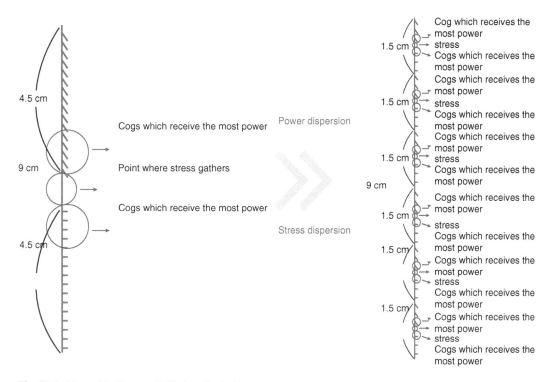

**Fig. 15.6**  N-cog lift. (Source: N-Finders Co, Ltd.)

Depending on the type of threads and the physician, there are various techniques. In this part, we deal with design, anesthesia, entry point, thread insertion, and cutting and finishing, which are the basics of thread lifting procedures. This chapter consists of useful techniques which are done most frequently in general and focuses on the methods for procedures using cog threads.

Depending on the physicians or conditions of patients, it is necessary to choose different techniques. Detailed techniques based on the types of the threads are dealt in 「Part VI. Techniques for Each Type」 and 「Part VII. Procedures for Each Part」.

Design is the most fundamental and crucial stage of thread lifting which determines the result of the procedures. As the direction and degree of sagging differ among people, it is recommendable to design accordingly. However, in practice, patients choose the type and number of the thread before procedures. In such case, it is difficult to achieve a good result. Through detailed designing, the best outcome can be achieved based on variable conditions. It is recommended that physicians try to pull the skin with various directions on patients' faces, and the key vector must be selected therefrom. To achieve a mutually satisfying result, sufficient communication is vital during the process. There are largely three common vectors used by the authors in cheek lifting.

- Vector which goes from the marionette line to the ear lobule.
    - This is called as the oblique vector in this chapter.
- Vector which passes the mandible-zygomatic arch-temple.
    - This is called as the vertical vector in this chapter.
- Vector which passes the nasolabial fold-zygomatic bone-hairline.
    - This is called as the nasolabial vector in this chapter.

## 16.1 Finding the Vector (Simulation) (Fig. 16.1)

Using one or both hands, we can predict the outcome of the procedure by pushing the skin in the direction you want to lift it. (The authors called this process as simulation.)

- (During consultation) Lifting simulation works better when the skin is lifted using two or three fingers or the palm rather than one finger. The patient should be educated that outcome varies depending on the type and the amount of threads. It can be explained to the patient that the difference between the simulation result of a finger and a palm is related to the number of threads used.
- Show expected outcome to the patient using the mirror.
- (During procedures) Once the type and the number of threads are chosen, find out a key vector that creates the best result through simulation.
- Draw horizontal lines/vertical lines/oblique lines which serve as reference lines.
- Mark the starting point and the ending point on the key vector line based on the length of threads.

## 16.2 Marking Reference Lines (Fig. 16.2)

1. Draw a horizontal line from the lateral canthus – ⓐ.

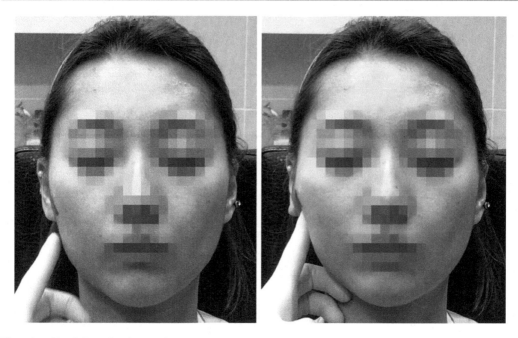

**Fig. 16.1** Simulation using fingers (finding adequate vectors)

**Fig. 16.2** Reference lines and basic vectors of design ●: locations of entry points at the time of inserting threads

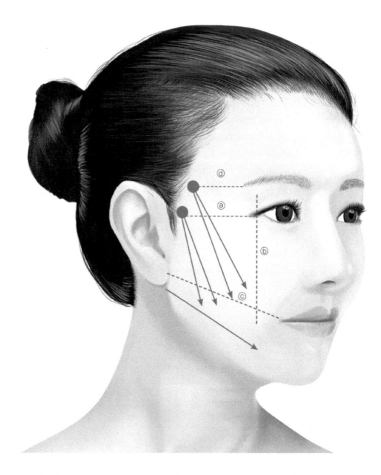

2. Draw a vertical line from the lateral canthus – ⓑ.
3. Draw a line which connects from the oral commissure to the lobule – ⓒ.
4. Draw a horizontal line from the end of the eyebrow – ⓓ.
   - Meaning of ⓐ: At the point where this line and the hairline meet, entry point can be marked for the nasolabial vector.
   - Meaning of ⓑ: When performing nasolabial lifting or marionette lifting, the hanging point does not need to be the desired area of pulling. Sufficient effect can be achieved even if the hanging point is not located medially to the line ⓑ.

**Tip!**
The reason that you don't need to make the hanging point medially over the line ⓑ.

- In case of threads with strong cogs, possibility of dimple is increased (see 「Part 9. Side Effects and Measures」).
- As the subcutaneous fat layer is very dense in this area, progressing a cannula requires much more force.
- As the subcutaneous fat layer is very dense in this area, the likelihood of tissue damage and blood vessel damage is higher.

- Meaning of ⓒ: In lifting sagged cheeks using the vertical vector, the hanging point doesn't need to reach to the desired area of pulling (as explained above, the desired area of pulling and the hanging point of the thread do not necessary coincide). Sufficient lifting can be achieved even if the ending point is not more below than the line ⓒ. This does not mean that the thread should never be inserted below this line. Moving approximately 1FB below the line ⓒ would be okay.

**Tip!**
The reason that it is not good to have the ending point much more below the line ⓒ.

- If the hanging point is placed near the jaw bone, threads with weak tensile strength may be cut, or the patient may experience pain when the mouth is opened widely.

- Meaning of ⓓ: When an entry point is made at the point where this reference line and the hairline meet (d'), precaution must be taken to avoid damage of the superficial temporal artery (STA). The STA runs more laterally to the hairline between a' and d' in most cases and drives more medially to the hairline after it passes d'. However, in some cases, it runs more medially to the hairline between a' and d'. Therefore, it's crucial to avoid STA damage by checking its pulse around the hairline while marking entry point prior to procedure.

## 16.3 Indicating Dangerous Areas

Indicate routes of the STA.

**Summary**
Importance of Thread Selection and Patient Selection

- Prior to designing, the type and amount of threads should be discussed with patients during consultation.
- If the patients have excessively high expectation or are not good candidates for thread lifting, it is not recommended.
- Therefore, it is advisable to select proper patients who will get a good level of results.

Importance of Design and Vectors

- Among all the process of thread lifting procedure, authors believe that designing process is the one which decisively influences the treatment outcome. Once patients are selected and the type of threads is chosen, the result of the procedure is expected to a certain extent. In general, the number of threads is determined during designing.
- During thread lifting training, designing of both sides is usually done by the trainer (the author). Thereafter, the author inserts the threads on the right side, and the trainee performs procedures on the other side.
- What do you think the outcome of the procedure would be? In conclusion, there is not much difference in the results from the right side and the left side. Of course, there is some difference in the occurrence of bleeding during procedures or dimples after procedures. However, if procedures are done after finding the key vector and designing, the results from both sides tend to be satisfactory.
- However, if designing is not done by the trainer but done directly by the trainee and procedures are performed (if the designing is not done with the key vector, but with an inappropriate vector), in most cases, they do not achieve the satisfactory result. Therefore, designing by finding the appropriate vector can be considered as a key step during the process.

## 17.1 Anesthesia Using Dental Lidocaine

### 17.1.1 Anesthesia Using the Dental Lidocaine (Figs. 17.1 and 17.2)

Inject locally in multiple areas.

**Advantages**
- It can be easily done by beginners.
- It can be done in much shorter time than anesthesia using cannulas.

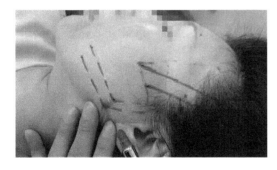

**Fig. 17.1** Anesthesia using the dental lidocaine

**Disadvantages**
- As needles are injected in multiple areas, bruising may occur.
- More painful than anesthesia using cannulas.

## 17.2 Anesthesia Using Cannulas

### 17.2.1 Anesthesia Using Cannulas (Tumescent Solutions or Lidocaine) (Figs. 17.3 and 17.4)

**Advantages**
- If anesthesia is performed using a dental lidocaine needle, dissatisfaction is sometimes experienced due to unexpected occurrence of bruising in anesthetic sites. However, if tumescent solution is injected through entry points using cannulas, bruising can be prevented nearly 100%.
- Less pain is experienced than in the anesthesia using the dental lidocaine.

**Disadvantages**
- It takes longer time than the anesthesia using the dental lidocaine.

© Springer Nature Singapore Pte Ltd. 2019
B. Kim et al., *The Art and Science of Thread Lifting*, https://doi.org/10.1007/978-981-13-0614-3_17

**Fig. 17.2** Anesthetic
sites using the dental
lidocaine

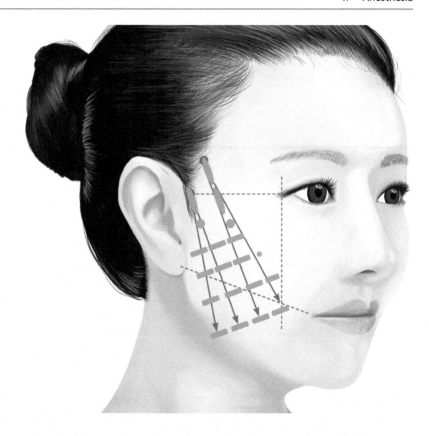

**Fig. 17.3** Anesthesia
using cannulas

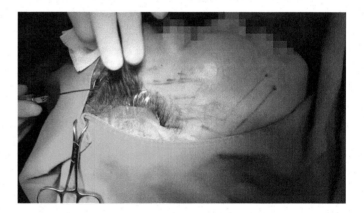

**Fig. 17.4** Route for
anesthesia using
cannulas

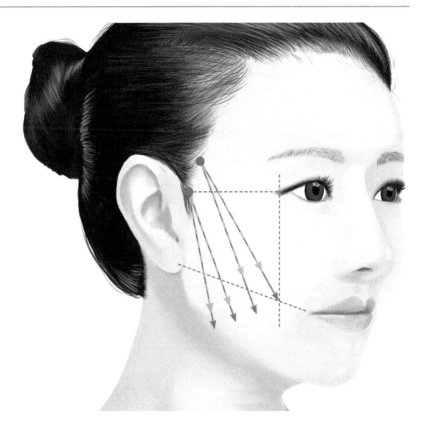

## 18.1 Location of Entry Point

Location of entry points varies depending on the direction of thread insertion (vector). In case of ⓐ and ⓑ vectors in Fig. 18.1, which are the most common vectors in lifting, the loca-

tions of entry points can be placed largely in three points.

1. To match the hairline
2. More inferomedial than the hairline
3. More superolateral than the hairline

**Fig. 18.1** Location of entry points. ●: entry point

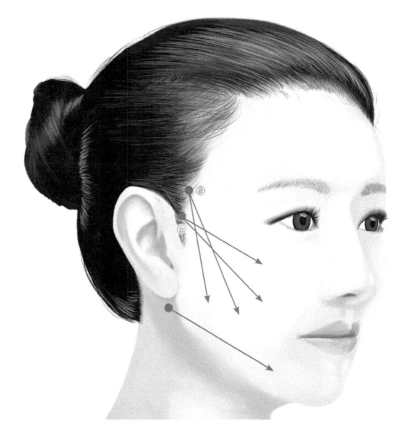

© Springer Nature Singapore Pte Ltd. 2019
B. Kim et al., *The Art and Science of Thread Lifting*, https://doi.org/10.1007/978-981-13-0614-3_18

## 18.2    Number of Entry Points

Once the vector and number of threads are decided, entry points should be made. There are two types.

1. Inserting one thread into one hole
2. Inserting multiple threads into one hole (most cases)

## 18.3    Selection of Entry Point Tools

There are two types of tools used in making entry points.

1. Disposable needle
2. Awl (Figs.18.2 and 18.3)

*Advantages in using awl*
- Low risk of bleeding (blunt)
- It creates large size entry point
  - If the hole is made too small due to the concern of bleeding, friction could occur while a cannula enters.

While making an entry point using the above tools, the correct layer it should penetrate is SQ layer. It is not necessary to penetrate the SMAS and muscles by deep puncture.

## 18.4    Cautions to Be Taken While Making Entry Point: Bleeding (Superficial Temporal Artery and Vein) (Figs.18.4 and 18.5)

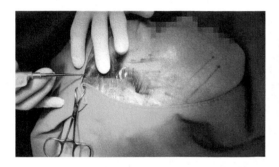

**Fig. 18.2**   Method of making entry points using awl

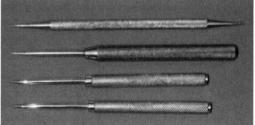

**Fig. 18.3**   Tools used in making entry points

**Fig. 18.4** Routes of vein (sentinel vein) and artery (superficial temporal artery) near the hairline – two vessels to be cautious of when making entry points

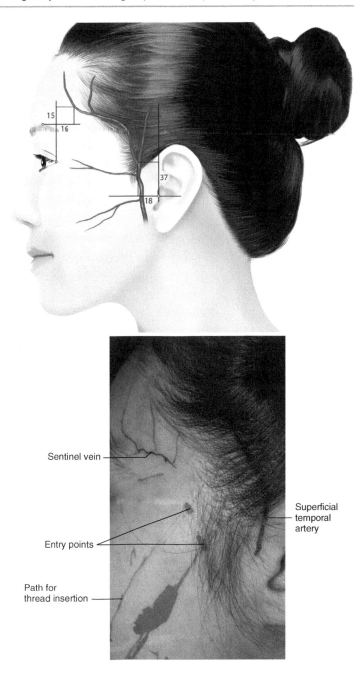

**Fig. 18.5** Route and depth of the superficial temporal artery near the hairline. Black arrow: After pinching and cutting the skin. STA is surrounded by the superficial temporal fascia. Red arrow: STA can be observed where the skin is intact. Blue dots: Original hairline. (Published with kind permission of © Wonsug Jung 2018. All rights reserved)

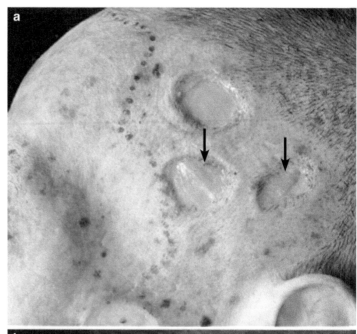

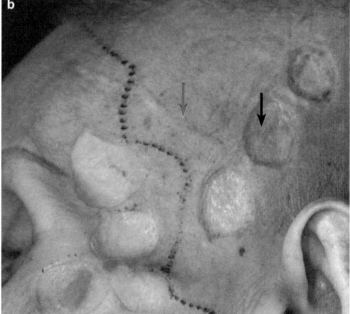

**Summary**
Solutions of Entry Point Bleeding

- Bleeding at entry point – In case of easily hemostasis (a few seconds ~ within 1 min)
  - Small-sized vessel injury.
  - Continue inserting the thread.
- Bleeding at entry point – In case that immediate hemostasis is not possible (2–3 min or longer)
  - This is a case of medium-sized vessel or branch of STA/STV damage. In such case, a new entry point must be made.
  - Generally, there is less blood vessel route in the medial side to the hairline. Try to make a new entry point by moving about 5 mm to the medial side.
- Bleeding after thread insertion
  - This is case of bleeding in the insertion route. This can occur if a blunt cannula is handled too roughly or a sharp needle is used.
  - Control bleeding and leave the thread as it is.
- Swelling from bleeding during cannula insertion
  - Sometimes swelling can occur due to bleeding in the cheek area during insertion of cannula (blunt/sharp). In such case, remove the cannula and do not insert the thread. Hemostasis must be applied for a long period.

## 18.5   Sterile Draping of Hairline

- Aseptic technique must be applied while making entry point along the hairline (see Fig. 23.7).
- Caution must be taken not to have the patient hair caught in the thread or entered into the entry point during procedures to avoid contamination.
- After the procedure ends, in general, skin tape is affixed on the entry point and removed after 2–3 days.

## 19.1 Various Techniques and Inserting Tools

*For beginners*
- Insertion using disposable cannula
  - Difference in blunt and sharp disposable cannulas
  - Difference in disposable cannula and surgical cannula

*For intermediate*
- Insertion of threads after inserting the cannula first
- Insertion using thread with needles at both ends of it

*For advanced*
- Temporal fascia anchoring (41 cm long) technique

### 19.1.1 Disposable Cannula (Blunt/ Sharp Cannula) (Fig. 19.1)

1. Difference in disposab le cannulas (blunt vs. sharp)

   *Blunt cannula (Fig. 19.2)*
   - Low risk of bleeding.
   - It is more unlikely to pass through tissues than sharp cannula.

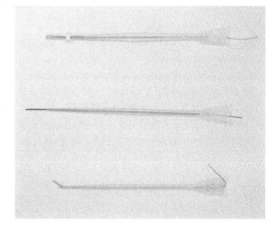

**Fig. 19.1** Disposable cannula – various products

*Sharp cannula*
- Higher risk of bleeding and penetration of the SMAS layer.
- If the depth is well adjusted, it can be passed with less force. (However, if the patient has severe acne scars, even sharp cannula can hardly pass the tissue.)

2. Difference in disposable and surgical cannulas (blunt/sharp)

   *Disposable cannula*
   - Duration of procedures can be shortened.
   - In proceeding with a cannula, it is difficult to reverse or take out from the entry point

after going forward. Once the cog thread is inserted into the tissues, the thread is immediately anchored, so that only the cannula can be pulled back. (Problems may occur if insertion depth is not well adjusted.) However, reversing is possible if only the proximal head of the cannula and thread is pressed by the thumb. While withdrawing the cannula, if any one of the cogs is inserted into tissue, further reversing is impossible. In such case, the cog would be anchored at inappropriate location, and then the thread and cannula must be removed.

*Surgical cannula (reusable cannula)*

• Each of the thread needs insertion of surgical cannula and subsequent insertion of thread into a sheath. So it requires longer treatment time.

• In proceeding with a cannula, going forward and reversing can be repeated. If the cannula is inserted at a depth that is not desired, it can be pulled back and be proceeded forward again.

## 19.2    Thread Insertion After Cannula Insertion (Figs. 19.3 and 19.4)

## 19.3    Temporal Anchoring (41 cm Long) U Pattern (Fig. 19.5)

## 19.4    Insertion Using a Thread with Needles at Both Ends. (Fig. 19.6)

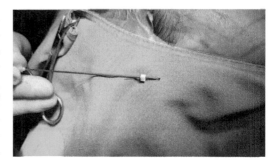

**Fig. 19.2**  Disposable cannula

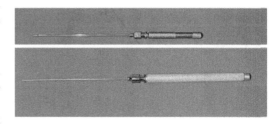

**Fig. 19.3**  Surgical cannula (reusable cannula). A guide needle with a blunt end is connected to the handle and the sheath which surrounds the outer surface covers the guide needle

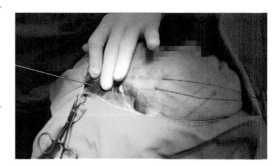

**Fig. 19.4**  Surgical cannula. As for the method of using a surgical cannula, insert the entire cannula first (guide needle + sheath), remove the guide needle, and then insert the thread into the sheath (In the figure, the long thread has already been inserted in a "U" shape)

**Fig. 19.5** Method of anchoring temporal fascia using long cannulas. (**a**) This is a process anchoring the temporal area using a curved needle for inserting long threads (details of this procedure are dealt with in 「Part 6–3 Technique of Fixing a Thread in the Temple」). (**b**) Tools needed for the procedure. From the left, sterile scissors, a long cannula set (17G), a temporal ring, an awl, cannula for anesthesia, and a design ruler

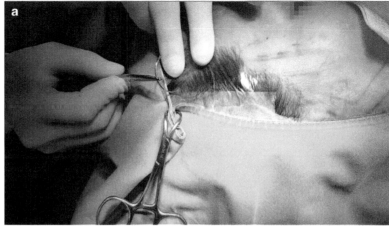

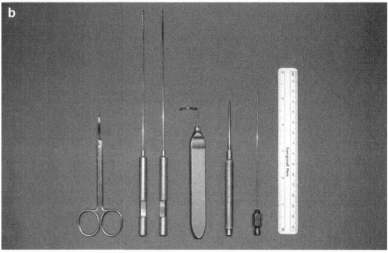

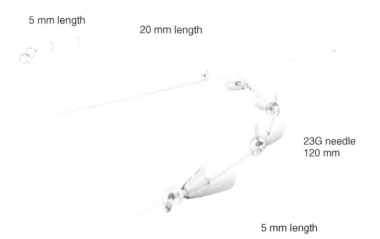

**Fig. 19.6** Thread for lifting which has needles attached to both ends. Although it is a long thread, a simple procedure can be performed without additional tools. Instead of cogs, cones exist between knots and they are bi-directional. For insertion, needles are attached to both ends of the thread (details are dealt with in 「Part 6–4 Technique of Inserting Bi-Directional Needle Threads」). (Source: Silhouette Soft®/SINCLAIR, https://www.sinclairpharma.com/silhouette-soft)

## 20.1 Removing Cannula

After a thread is inserted and its cannula is being removed, the skin is to be pressed upward using the opposite fingers. (Press upward the skin surface of thread insertion area in a desired direction.)

## 20.2 Cutting

### 20.2.1 Cutting While Pulling the Thread

1. Precaution

    If pulling of the threads is not consistent that just one thread is pulled strongly, the middle of the bi-directional thread which is strongly pulled is elevated, and the remaining threads inserted in the area are not elevated. Finally focal protrusion/depression can occur. This can cause patient's dissatisfaction.

It is important for the physician to keep in mind that all threads need to be pulled evenly.

2. Prevention of focal bulging/depression
    - When a thread is pulled, an assistant should press approximately 2–3 cm below the entry point and then cut with sterile scissors while pushing the skin.
    - If it occurs in the zygomatic arch level, the likelihood of dissatisfaction increases due to the widening of the cheekbones. So design must be done in a way that the middle point of the bi-directional thread does not coincide with the zygomatic arch level.

### 20.2.2 Cutting While Pushing the Skin

Cut while slightly pushing the skin and then embed the tip of the thread in the SQ.

# Part VI
# Techniques for Various Types of Thread

# Technique Using a Mono-thread

21

Summary of histologic changes after PDO thread insertion

- Newly developed fibrous connective tissue
- Merging with existing fibrous connective tissue
- Tissue contraction by myofibroblast
- Increased capillary vessel size
- Fat cell denaturation

## 21.1 Mono-thread Insertion

From a theoretical perspective, it is difficult to see mono-threads having good lifting effects. Basically, as the concept of the fixing point is not clear and the theoretical basis for the creation of direction is thought to result from contraction of the subcutaneous fat tissues, the effect would be weak. The authors will talk about their thoughts more in detail later. In such case, there is some difference in effect, consistency, and duration of the procedures depending on the physicians. However, based on author's experience, it is possible to make good outcomes when a sufficient number of threads are inserted using adequate methods. This technique has been used for a long time and is still being used widely.

Theoretical explanations about the above technique are expressed in Figs. 21.1 and 21.2. When threads are inserted into two sites, tissues are pulled to more thread inserted side. We will review about such outcome results later in detail.

The theoretical basis is deduced from the mono-thread insertion based on the tissue experimental results shown in the article <Tissue changes over time after polydioxanone thread insertion: An animal study with pigs> by Jung Hyun Yoon et al. Histological changes from PDO thread insertion are summarized in the following.

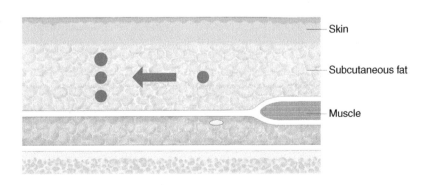

**Fig. 21.1** Changes after inserting a mono-thread. The past theory explains that direction is created from less insertion point to more insertion point

© Springer Nature Singapore Pte Ltd. 2019
B. Kim et al., *The Art and Science of Thread Lifting*, https://doi.org/10.1007/978-981-13-0614-3_21

103

Namely, the effect of the mono-thread insertion is attaching the sagged tissues inward rather than pulling the tissue with direction.

Considering the aging change at the level of fat, fibrous tissue, and skin with the histologic change from thread insertion, it can be deduced that the following results can be obtained:

- Due to the effects of fat denaturation from insertion of mono-threads and effects of proliferation and contraction of fibrotic tissues, the size of the bulging fat decreases. As a result, there is a tightening effect in which the face sticks inward.
- New fibrotic tissues are created and connected to the pre-existing surrounding fibrotic tissues. In conclusion, the structure of the subcutaneous fibrous connective tissues becomes dense and strong.
- Through the myofibroblast formed around inserted threads, contraction effects of tissues

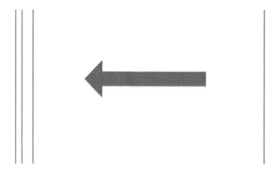

**Fig. 21.2** Changes after inserting a mono-thread. The past theory explains that direction is created from less insertion point to more insertion point

occur. This can explain the effect of pulling the sagged face skin inward.
- It can be expected that the skin environment will be improved by the findings that the size of the capillaries increase.

In the end, effect of mono-thread insertion can be expected to be caused by contraction of fat tissue, strengthening of fibrous connective tissue, and improvement of the dermal environment.

Based on the tissue slide opinion of the study done by Jung Hyun Yoon et al., only in the tissues which are nearby the threads are seen to denature fat. However, as the amount of the subcutaneous fat in the face itself is not much and due to additional effects (proliferation and merging effect of fibrotic tissues), some beneficial effects may be made from fat denaturation and contraction of fibrotic tissues through the PDO insertion. Based on objective index on the lifting effects, we plan to conduct researches which evaluate the results quantitatively using such index.

## 21.2  Difference in Changes from the Mono-thread Technique

The outcome of discussions with various doctors about how deep threads are inserted in clinical practices and why they are performed in such way is as follows.

**Fig. 21.3** Method of inserting a mono-thread. Method of inserting threads: wave form insertion in order to increase the contact area with the subcutaneous fat layer

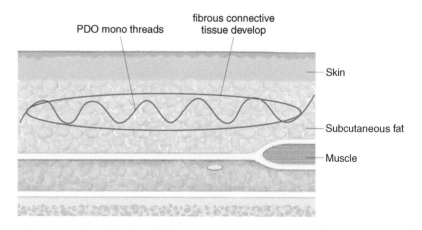

In general, the opinion is that to shrink the sagged fat layer, a thread is to be inserted into the subcutaneous fat, and to pull the sagged skin, a thread is to be inserted closely attached to the subdermis area. Considering the changes after inserting the PDO, we think this is an adequate technique for procedures. To reduce the fat layer, it seems that inserting deeply while increasing contacts with the fat layer as much as possible would be effective, and to cause changes to the dermis, we think it would be useful to locate the thread closely to the dermal layer.

The study which discovers the difference in the relative histologic changes based on the depth of the PDO insertion is thought to be able to bring an important result in establishing a theoretical background for the thread lifting techniques in the future. It is also necessary to study the pattern of tissue change according to the shape and thickness of thread.

## 21.3   Explanations About the Mechanism

### 21.3.1   Method of the Mono-thread Technique: Neckline (Fig. 21.4)

- For more definition of the jawline, insert the PDO mono-threads above and below the jawline making sure they are also parallel to the jawline.
- Create a jawline by causing contraction of the fat layer and conglutination of fibrotic tissues.
- If the PDO is inserted like a wave passing in and out of the subcutaneous fat layer and the SMAS layer, tissue contraction may be expected in a wider area as the threads go through the process of fibrosis while they melt. In clinical practice, the method of inserting the threads by moving the top and bottom parts of the fat layer rather than simply inserting was once popular.

**Fig. 21.4** Mono-thread procedure technique. Method of inserting threads above and below along the jawline

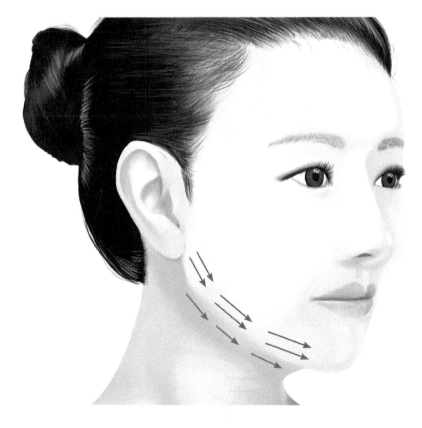

### 21.3.2 Mono-thread Technique: Jowl
(Fig. 21.5)

- The anatomical explanations about the reason for bulging of the inner cheek area are as follows:
  - Due to an empty space between the risorius m. and zygomaticus major, the SMAS is not continuous, and an empty space is created. Deep fat tissues which are stretched from aging push and come out mainly through this area.
- The mechanism of procedures on the inner cheek using the PDO mono-threads is using the effect of fat denaturation, fibrosis effect, and tissue contraction effect of the PDO.
- On one hand, in case of using a hard PDO twister-type thread in a spring form, an effect of pressing fat which sticks out like by causing the muscles to cover fat in this area may be expected. In reality, the twister-type PDO in a

spring form is expected to have an effect of pressing tissues and volumizing effects and is used in various areas.

### 21.3.3 Mono-thread Technique: Frontal Cheek and Nasolabial Fold (Fig. 21.7)

- Drooping frontal cheek areas are elements which aggravate the nasolabial folds. Through inserting mono-threads in the area where the frontal cheek droops above the nasolabial fold, conglutination of fibrotic tissues and contraction of fat cells may be expected.
- As a result, there is an effect of pushing the bulging frontal cheek in slightly.
- If a slightly thicker and harder spring-type monofilament is inserted from the cheek to over the nasolabial fold area, there is an effect

**Fig. 21.5** Mono-thread technique. Method of performing procedures to cause shrinking of the jowl area

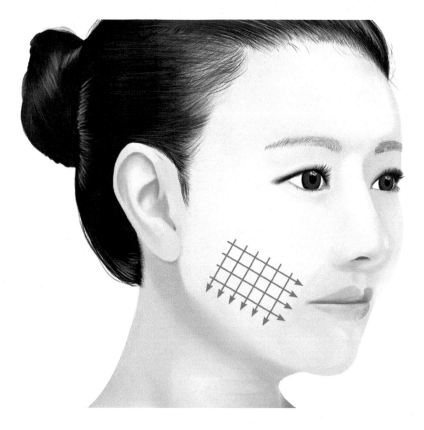

**Fig. 21.6** Anatomical mechanism of the fat bulging inner cheek. (Published with kind permission of © Kwan-Hyun Youn 2018. All rights reserved)

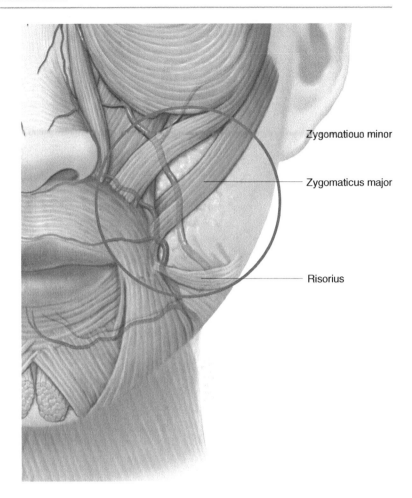

Zygomatiouo minor

Zygomaticus major

Risorius

of reducing the frontal cheek by pressing with force the hard PDO thread.

### 21.3.4 Mono-thread Technique: Temples (Fig. 21.8)

Due to aging, wrinkles and sagging are formed around the eye area. The fundamental treatment would be the forehead lifting surgery or eyelid surgery, but a simple procedure using mono-thread lifting is also possible. Of course, the effect does not reach that of surgical treatment.

If hard PDO threads in a spring form are inserted in a radial shape in the temple area, it can be seen that the eyebrows are slightly lifted.

As the PDO in a spring form is hard as well as having small volume, it plays a role of volumiz-

ing and lifting the sagged eye areas and the temple areas. However, the effect and duration are questionable. Comparative clinical experiments seem necessary.

The most advanced thread lifting technique is anchoring the threads in the temple area using long various tools. This requires a technique (know-how) of pulling with long threads with fixing points making around the temples.

Classification of thread lifting techniques:

1. Short-thread technique (QT lift) – disposable cannula/needle
2. Long-thread technique(QT lift) – long cannula
3. Technique using a thread with needles attached in both sides (Silhouette Soft®)

**Fig. 21.7** Mono-thread
technique – frontal
cheek and nasolabial

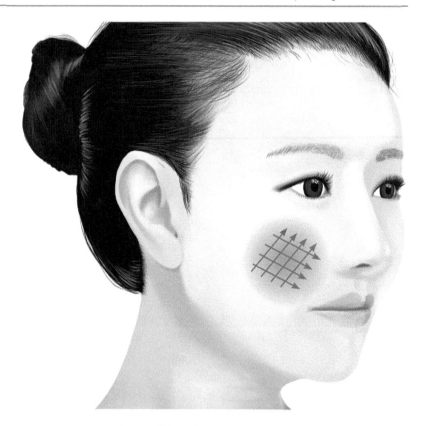

**Fig. 21.8** Techniques
for the mono-thread of
the spring-type temples.
Insert threads into the
subcutaneous fat layer in
a radial shape. A
volumizing effect with
lifting effect can be
expected

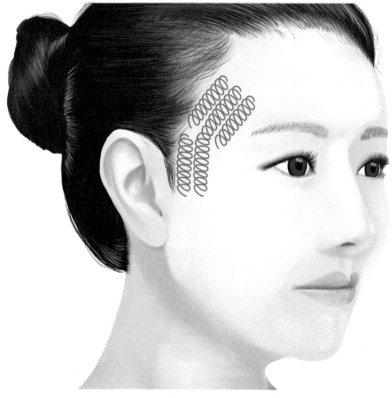

## 22.1 Unidirectional Cog Thread

After inserting the cogs to be hung on tissues, pull them in one direction. The lifting effect is maintained only if the fixing point of thread is made in anyway.

However, based on the structure and mechanism of the thread, it is difficult to maintain the lifting effect (Fig. 22.1). Nowadays, this type of thread is used for limited cases.

## 22.2 Spike

Threads in a spike form are used for fixing after performing lifting using bi-directional cog threads, etc. first. Among various techniques of thread lifting, after dissecting the layer to which the thread is to be inserted, if the thread in a spike form is inserted into such layer after adjusting the up-and-down direction well (Fig. 22.2), it plays the function of fixing the dissected and dislocated plane. When lifting through plane dissection is performed, spike-form thread is useful rather than cog thread.

The following matters need to be considered in performing a spike thread procedure:

- It is advisable to insert for fixing in the area where tissues are dislocated through dissection.
- It is advisable to insert accurately on the surface where the upper board and the lower board are separated through dissection, and the direction of cogs is very important. After accurately finding out the direction of lifting, the spike thread must be inserted. The pulled direction and the lying direction of cogs in the upper side of the thread must coincide (Fig. 22.3).
- If it is inserted into an opposite direction, fixing does not occur and it slips, not stabilizing the pulled tissues. Surely, this will not be able to maintain the lifting effect.

Through Fig. 22.3, it can be seen well which side the top and bottom of spike cogs must be. Lifting can be maintained only if the spike cog is inserted in the direction which prevents driving

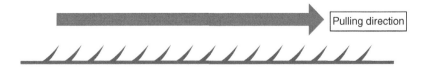

Pulling direction

**Fig. 22.1** Unidirectional cog. It can be fixed after pulling tissues in one direction

© Springer Nature Singapore Pte Ltd. 2019
B. Kim et al., *The Art and Science of Thread Lifting*, https://doi.org/10.1007/978-981-13-0614-3_22

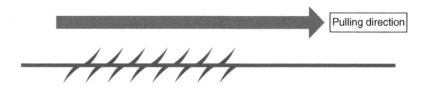

**Fig. 22.2** Spike thread. Rather than the function of pulling tissues, it stabilizes already pulled tissues, and the up-and-down direction is important

**Fig. 22.3** Right insertion direction; pulled tissues can be stabilized

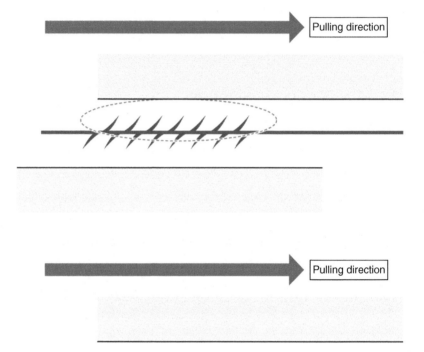

**Fig. 22.4** Wrong insertion direction; this cannot stabilize the pulled tissues

which returns in the direction that is opposite from the pulled direction.

On the other hand, based on Fig. 22.4, if the direction of cogs can't prevent the movement of the tissue to return to the original position, pulled tissue would be slipped. Therefore, when spike threads are used, direction is very important.

## 22.3  Zigzag Method

The mechanism of the bi-directional zigzag cog method is as follows (Fig. 22.5):

- The cog thread of zigzag method is largely used for fixing pulled tissues after performing lifting rather than for lifting itself.

- After lifting procedure using bi-directional cog threads, to prevent side effects like sinking, zigzag threads are sometimes inserted supplementary.

## 22.4 Bi-directional Cog

### 22.4.1 Understanding Bi-directional Cogs

Bi-directional cogs consist of forward cogs which play the role of pulling and reverse cogs which play the role of fixing the pulled tissues not to go down (Fig. 22.6). In the end, it has effects of lifting the tissues in both sides to the middle part without any cog.

It has better effect than unidirectional cogs.

As seen in the figure, the accurate function of bi-directional cog threads is not to pull in one direction but to gather in the middle part (Figs. 22.7 and 22.8). Namely, it can be understood as a method of pulling both sides to the middle area. If design and procedures are performed with well understanding of this mechanism, a good result can be expected.

By using such characteristics of the bi-directional cogs, the sunken facial area can be adjusted (Fig. 22.9). If there are adequate design and technical support for the facial shape, lifting in any form is possible.

### 22.4.2 Experiment on Actual Bi-directional Cogs

1. After preparing a wide area in the subcutaneous fat layer of pork, areas below the muscle layer were removed.
2. After inserting a 19 G bi-directional cog thread to the skin perpendicularly, progress was made in a consistent depth through the subcutaneous layer by changing the direction horizontally.
3. After removing the cannula, the cog thread was pulled.
4. Changes were observed thereafter (Fig. 22.10).

**Fig. 22.5** Zigzag method (multi-bi-directional cog). It stabilizes pulled tissues in the middle

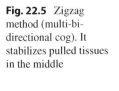

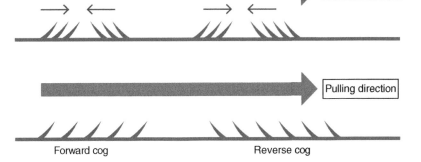

**Fig. 22.6** Bi-directional cog

Forward cog          Reverse cog

**Fig. 22.7** After simple insertion

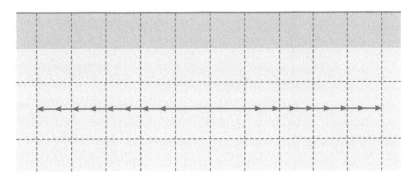

**Fig. 22.8** Pulled after insertion. If this is used wrongly, it can be a cause of side effects

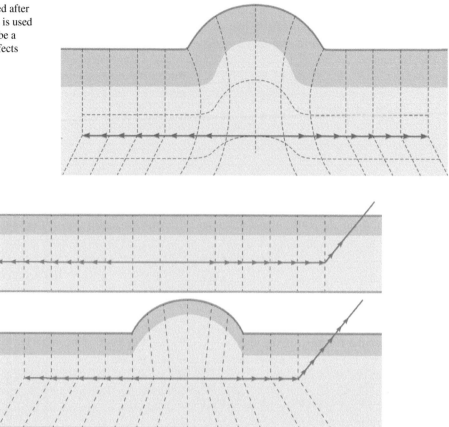

**Fig. 22.9** Actual practice with bi-directional cogs. By causing the tissues in the middle part to be gathered, the bi-directional cogs show lifting effects. In actual practice, it is also important to understand the function of the area where the cog thread enters subcutaneously. The entry point area of the thread inevitably passes beneath the der- mis; the cog thread tends to be hung hard at that point. Lifting effects can be maximized by using the effect of gathering tissues to the middle area and the effect of cogs in the opposite direction of the cog thread hanging in the bottom of the dermis well

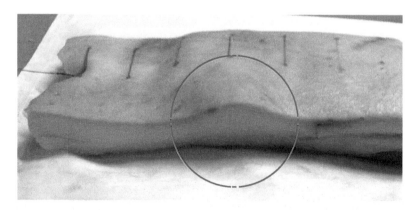

**Fig. 22.10** Traction test of bi-directional cogs. The appear- ance after inserting the bi-directional cog thread into the sub- cutaneous layer and pulling in one direction can be seen. Although it is slightly distant from the thread entry site, when it is seen through a cutting surface, it can be seen that the subcutaneous fat layer that coincides with the middle area of the cogs is gathered and inflated. If the procedures are performed after understanding the mechanism well, it has the effect of gathering tissues as well as the effect of lift- ing, namely, the effect of volumizing through redisposition

### 22.4.2.1 Angle Technique Using Bi-directional Cogs

The angle technique can be understood as an expansion of bi-directional cogs. As mentioned previously, bi-directional cogs create lifting effects by repositioning tissues to the middle where there is no cog. In case of the angle technique, by causing the angle to be slightly bent, rather than in straight line, it is a method of causing the tissues inside the bent angle to gather (Fig. 22.11).

It has effects of adjusting sinking, together with lifting effects, and various designs are possible.

Insert the cannula with threads and proceed (Fig. 22.12), then deflect the direction at angle point, and insert to the end.

Remove the cannula from the skin and pull the thread to make the tissue inflated.

### 22.4.2.2 V Technique (Bending and Fixing)

### 22.4.2.3 Methods of Tying Cog Threads

Tying method means tying of the cog thread at the fixing point. A thickened tie enters inside the skin thereafter and acts as a stronger fixing point than simple cog thread insertion using uni- or bi-directional cogs.

### 22.4.2.4 X-Cross Technique

To strengthen and maintain the lifting effect, it is important to utilize reverse directional cogs. In general, remaining cogs are removed after the desired length of insertion. In some case, a significant amount of reverse directional cogs is cut out.

To optimize the lifting effect, it is important to vitalize the function of reverse cogs. In such case, without removing the remaining cogs, the method of pushing them toward the opposite direction can be used (Fig. 22.13). In addition, by tying the middle part of the cog thread, it can be combined with the method of making one more area which can act as a fixing point (Fig. 22.14). By using the two skills together, it is a method of strengthening the function of the fixing points (Fig. 22.15).

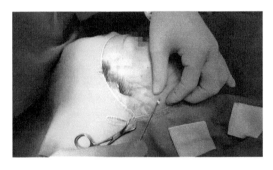

**Fig. 22.12** Techniques of bi-directional cog thread – insertion of angle technique

**Fig. 22.11** Bi-directional cog thread technique – concept of angle technique

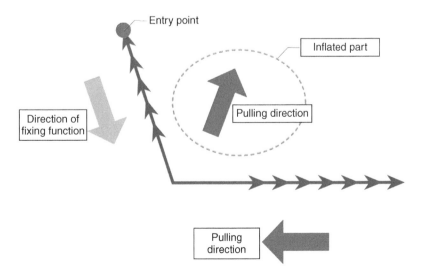

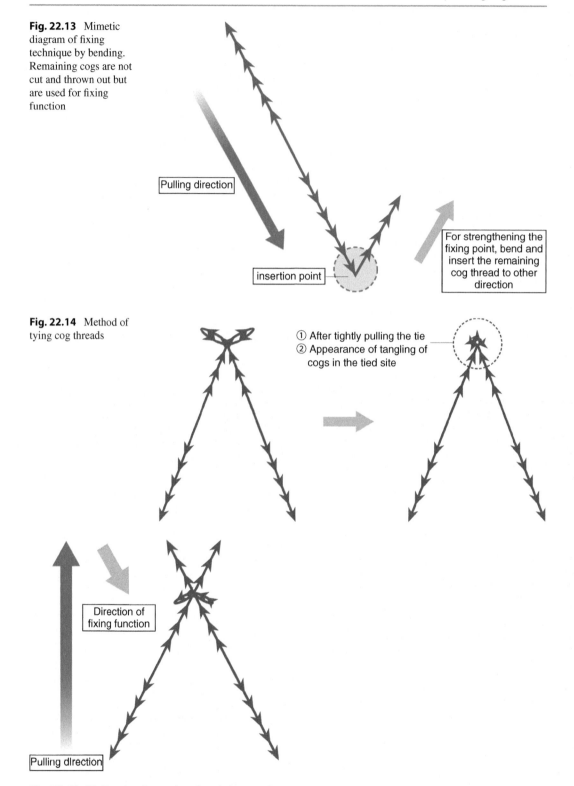

**Fig. 22.13** Mimetic diagram of fixing technique by bending. Remaining cogs are not cut and thrown out but are used for fixing function

Pulling direction

insertion point

For strengthening the fixing point, bend and insert the remaining cog thread to other direction

**Fig. 22.14** Method of tying cog threads

① After tightly pulling the tie
② Appearance of tangling of cogs in the tied site

Direction of fixing function

Pulling direction

**Fig. 22.15** Bi-directional cog thread technique – the X-cross technique concept has the advantage of using the remaining opposite directional cogs without having to throw them out

## 23.1 Mechanisms

The difference between lifting of the anchoring method and others using a mono-thread or cog thread is that it can make a strong fixing point.

It is ideal to anchor a thread in the fascia of the anchoring site (Fig. 23.1). If the thread is anchored in the subcutaneous fat layer, the fixing force is weak. Understanding the changes in tissues that occur when pinch manipulation is performed at the temple area, the thread can be reliably anchored to the fascia layer. The thread should be appropriately anchored to the temple area fascia by pinch manipulation where there is no large vessels. After the anchoring is done properly, the remaining thread is inserted to the subcutaneous layer and exits out to perform the lifting procedure.

The pulled skin is placed in a folded state at the anchored area (Fig. 23.2). And it is maintained by cogs of thread. The instant result is stronger than the mono-thread method and the simple cog thread lifting procedures. The longevity is determined by the strength of the cogs, efficiency of the cogs, sustainability of threads, and expertise of the physician.

**Summary**
Design Method (Fig. 23.3)

1. Facial landmarks and reference line
   ⓐ Horizontal line at the lateral canthus
   ⓑ Perpendicular line at the lateral canthus
   ⓒ Line connecting from the oral commissure to the lobule
   ⓓ Horizontal line from the end of the eyebrow

2. Mark a reference line inside the hairline
   ⓔ Perpendicular line at the center of the tragus
   ⓕ Temporal crest: it appears simultaneously with masseter muscle contraction

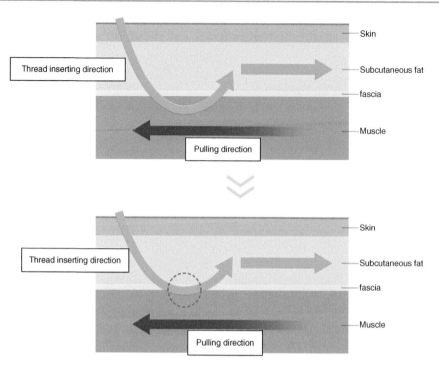

**Fig. 23.1** Fascia anchoring method. This shows the mechanism of hanging the thread in the fascia and making a fixing point

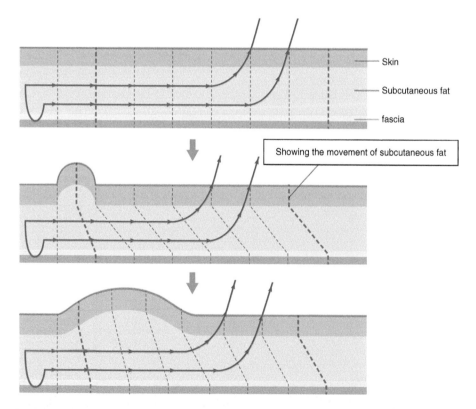

**Fig. 23.2** Understanding of lifting mechanisms about fascia anchoring method; pulled tissues gather in at some point between the fixing point and the exit

**Fig. 23.3** Design of the fascia anchoring method

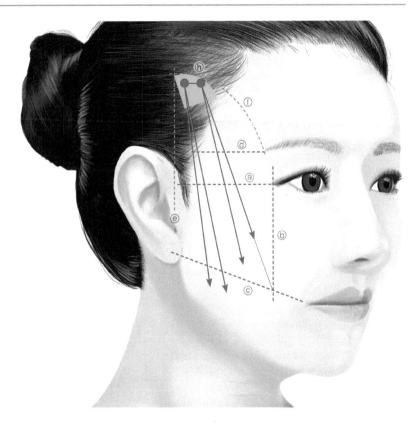

3. Entry point
   Assuming that the semicircle located from approximately two finger breadth from the crossing point of ⓒ and ⓕ is ⓑ, it is convenient to set an entry point therein. If you make an entry point higher than this, it is difficult to handle the cannula because of the curved surface of the skull. If lower than this, you may cause damage to the anterior branch of the STA (superficial temporal artery. see Fig. 23.4) resulting in massive bleeding.

**Summary**

Cautions    to    be    Considered    during Designing

1. Prevention of "slanted eyes" and sentinel vein rupture
   If the innermost thread is near the lateral canthus, the lateral canthus may be lifted after the procedure. In some cases with young patients, they desire lifting the lateral canthus, but patients in their mid- to elder ages generally consider lifting of the lateral canthus to be unnatural. Therefore, it is necessary to explain about the lateral canthus rising, and if that is not desired, the design of thread pathway should not be done so close to the lateral canthus. It is advisable to distance at least two finger breadths away from the lateral canthus (arrows in Fig. 23.5). When designing as above, it will not overlap the running of sentinel vein).

2. Prevention of aggravation of fine wrinkles under the eyes
   With the rising of the lateral canthus, when the infraorbital skin is pulled, the fine wrinkles below the eyes may appear deeper. This can be prevented to a certain extent by designing the thread to pass through two finger breadths away from the lateral canthus. During designing, by

actually pulling the skin with the finger, check whether the under-eye wrinkles become deeper together with whether the lateral canthus lifts or not.

3. Passing the sunken cheek must be prevented

4. Cautions to be taken at the area of frequent dimples

When the exit of the thread is located medially, it is advisable to stay within the crossing points of the blue-dotted line (limit line) as shown in Fig. 23.6 ③ and ④. If the exit is medial passing the crossing point, the lifting effect of mouth sagging may become better, but due to the occurrence of dimples, patient's satisfaction level is more likely to decrease.

5. STA point to be cautious of −1

When designing the pathway of the outermost thread, do not design in the space between the tragus and inner one finger breadth where the pulse of STA is most strong. It is advisable to design at least 1.5 -2 finger breadth away from center of the tragus (arrow of Fig. 23.5 ). If the distance is closer than this, the likelihood of STA damage becomes high, and also, there may be claim of "Łwrinkling of the skin in front of the ear"Ł after the procedure (patients with skin laxity).

6. STA point to be cautious of −2

The entry point should be within range ⓑ. In some cases, an anterior or parietal branch of STA may run within that range. Before you make entry points, you must check whether you feel a pulse.

**Summary**

Hairline preparation and draping.

1. Hairline preparation

Either cut few pieces of hair with scissors or shave using a shaver. In preparing the hairline, all hair in the opposite area to the progression direction as well as the progression direction must be prepared.

Preparing the hair pieces to the minimum extent is necessary for the easy posttreatment management. Unexpected bleeding can occur severely in some cases in anchoring threads in the temporal areas. In such case, we must change the anchoring location inevitably. Considering this, it is advisable to prepare the hairline enough to allow anchoring twice.

2. Fixing (Fig. 23.7)

Prepare the nearby hairline using the Fixomer, Tegaderm®, hairpins, rubber bands, 3M, etc. If procedures are performed without this step completely, it would interfere with thread insertion a lot. Moreover, if hair gets into the entry point, it can cause folliculitis. Therefore, it is advisable to clean and prepare the hairline prior to the procedure.

3. Disinfecting

In order to prevent foreign substances from getting into the cannula during insertion, areas which touch the cannula or all areas which can touch the cannula, including the hair, must be strictly disinfected.

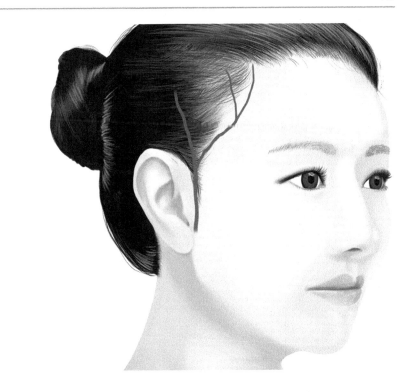

**Fig. 23.4** Blood vessels to be cautious in designing the fascia anchoring method – STA (superficial temporal artery)

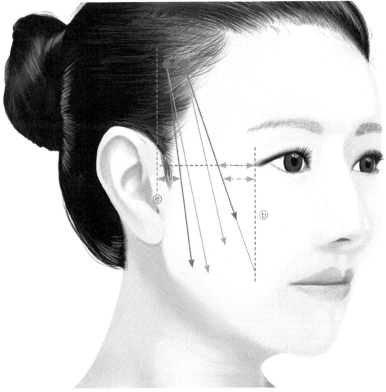

**Fig. 23.5** Cautions to be taken in designing the fascia anchoring method – "slanted eyes"

**Fig. 23.6** Cautions to be taken in designing the fascia anchoring method – area of frequent dimples

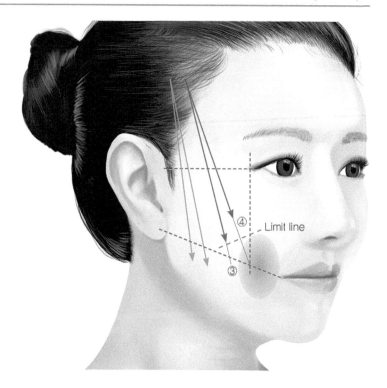

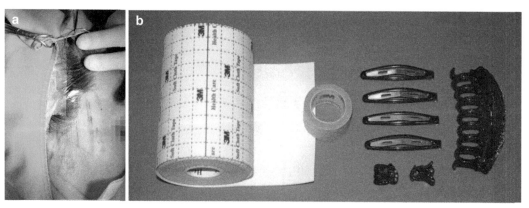

**Fig. 23.7** Preparations for the fascia anchoring method – draping and preparing the hairline. (**a**) Showing of attaching a sterile Tegaderm®. (**b**) Tools needed to prepare the hairline

## 23.2 Insertion Method

### 23.2.1 Design

### 23.2.2 Anesthesia Method

1. Anesthesia of entry and exit points – needle
   - It is advisable to anesthetize the entry and exit points using lidocaine (1: 100,000) which includes epinephrine. If the exit is not anesthetized, bruising can occur due to the dermal plexus bleeding.

2. Anesthesia of thread progression route
   1. Injection of tumescent solution or lower-concentration lidocaine using a cannula
      - Proper anesthesia allows smooth cannula insertion during thread lifting. Using very long and thin one can reduce pain, but it is difficult to maintain consistent driving depth and easy bends during progression; an adequate thickness is recommended (diameter of 0.9–1.0 mm).

- In lieu of a cannula, there is also a method of injecting anesthetic agents conveniently into various points of thread pathway using needle and dental lidocaine, but it has some disadvantages.
  - As anesthesia does not occur as desired, it may require additional anesthesia during thread insertion.
  - If needles are inserted in various places, due to dermal plexus bleeding, a likelihood of bruising increases.
2. Lidocaine local anesthesia using needles
  - In the long-thread lifting procedure, the thread passes through the subcutaneous fat layer. However, as the subcutaneous fat layer is not an area where pain senses are well developed, pain is minimal in general when driving the subcutaneous fat layer except some specific area (mainly vessel crossing area).
  - Using this, a small amount of lidocaine is sometimes injected using a needle into the driving route to anesthetize.
    - Advantages are that less swelling occurs after the procedure, the procedure becomes simple, and the depth of driving can be learned through finding out patient's pain.
    - On the other hand, compared to anesthetizing the driving route using a cannula, patients can feel pain in the interim and become anxious.

## 23.3   Entry Point and Anchoring

### 23.3.1   Tools for Entry Points

1. Awl
  - It is suggested to use an awl than a needle.
  - Advantages
    1. Risk of bleeding is low (blunt).
    2. If the hole is made small as a result of concern for bleeding, the friction causes difficulty in advancing the cannula. By using an awl, a hole with a sufficient size can be procured. Progressing a cannula becomes convenient.

### 23.3.2   Anchoring Tools

1. Needle
2. Temporal ring (Fig. 23.8)
  - Advantages over a needle
    1. Likelihood of bleeding decreases significantly.
    2. Less chance to develop a dimple at entry point

### 23.3.3   Depth and Direction of Anchoring Point

There are various opinions as follows:

- Fixing at the periosteum
- Fixing at the deep temporal fascia: theoretically
- Fixing at the superficial temporal fascia

> **Tip!**
> In some cases where SQ tissues at the anchoring point are too loose
> In the process of pulling the thread after the insertion, in some cases, loose SQ tissues cannot attach and hold to the thread, and the thread is dragged down from the anchoring point. Even if the SQ tissues are relatively dense, if the physician pulls the thread too strongly, the same can occur. Therefore, an assistant must press the anchoring point with the fingers when the thread is pulled.

- Fixing at the deep SQ
An entry point can be located in the line of the temporal crest (viz., much more above than the ⓑ area in Fig. 23.3). In such case, there are advantages of reducing bleeding which can occur during temporal fascia anchoring and anchoring to more solid tissues (periosteum). However, differently from the structure of the skull of Westerners, as in many cases, Asians have triangular skull (not trigonocephaly, but the skull is more developed than the size of the face), it is not easy for a cannula to drive along the curve at a consistent depth.

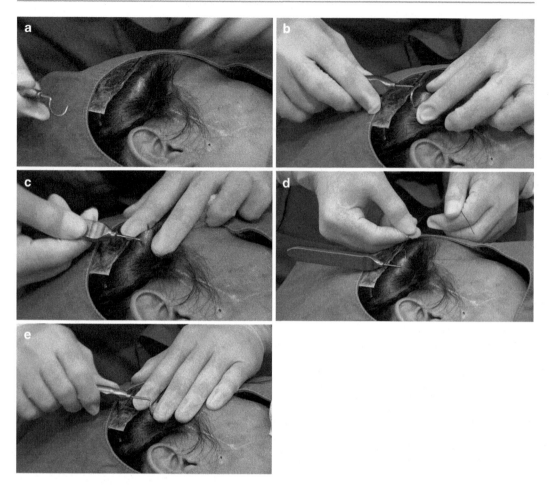

**Fig. 23.8** Tools for the fascia anchoring method (temporal ring). (**a**) Taking a temporal ring of which the end looks semicircular. (**b**) Between the two entry points, insert one side first (in this case, the two entry points can be made in advance using an awl or a needle). (**c**) After anchoring by revolving the temporal ring, exit to the opposite entry point (causes the ring to come out partially to the extent of exposing the hole in the temporal ring). (**d**) Put the thread in the hole at the end of the ring. (**e**) Take out the temporal ring by revolving again in the direction opposite from the insertion

---

**Tip!**
Direction of Anchoring

  Based on Michael A. Carron et al., when anchoring is performed in the fascia area of the temporalis muscle, it has been discovered that the resistance against the pulling power is stronger in the horizontal method than in the vertical method (1.9 vs 5.01, tearing force kg/cm).

**Summary**
Measures for Bleeding While Anchoring: Long Threads

1. Bleeding after anchoring with a needle
   • Injury to small blood vessels
     Bleeding may show due to damage of small blood vessels from a sharp needle, after the passing of the needle or the thread, but if it stopped by pressuring, the inserted thread may continue to proceed.

- When vessel penetration is suspected

  In some cases, almost no bleeding occurs after a needle pass, but significant bleeding occurs after the thread is put on the needle and then anchored, resulting in swelling in the entry point area. This may be caused by passing of a sharp needle through the middle of a thick blood vessel. As it was fine when the needle passes initially, physician believes that it will stop bleeding soon. But, despite the long pressure, hemostasis is not easy. This is because vessel damage is aggravated when a thread penetrates a blood vessel. In such case, it is advisable to cut the middle of the bi-directional thread and remove it. Thereafter, pressure for a sufficient period to stop bleeding and perform the procedure again with another entry point elsewhere.

2. Bleeding after anchoring with a temporal ring

   As the ring is thicker than a needle, even an injury occurs during anchoring process and blood will not emerge at the entry point immediately. After putting the thread and passing, bleeding shows. If bleeding does not easily stop, in such case also, the thread needs to be removed and discarded.

   → Differently from a needle, a temporal ring is thicker, forming a tunnel through anchoring. After anchoring, rather than putting the thread right away, take out the temporal ring, and check whether there is any bleeding in the place where it passed. If there is no bleeding, put the thread back after inserting the temporal ring again to the preformed tunnel. If there is bleeding, anchor to another point after hemostasis. If such method is used, the cases of removing threads due to bleeding after anchoring with a temporal ring can be reduced.

3. Blood vessel damage from cogs

   As a thread drives, blood vessel damages may occur also from cogs. However, in such case, bleeding can be stopped easily and the inserted thread may continue to proceed.

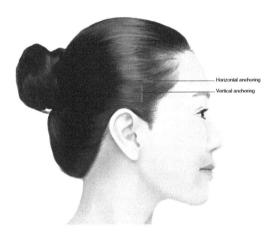

Horizontal anchoring
Vertical anchoring

### 23.3.4 Side Effects: Prevention and Treatments for Headache

Headaches may occur when fixing is done on the fascia.

1. There is no need to prescribe NSAID or Tylenol as a routine, but through listening to the medical history prior to the procedure, if a medical history of temporal area headache is present, it is advisable to prescribe this as a preventive measure.

2. If a headache occurs after the procedure, in some cases, a painkiller would not solve it, but the headache is cured through injecting botulinum toxin. Currently, botulinum toxin has obtained an FDA approval as having preventive effects for chronic recurrent migraine. However, based on the meta-analysis by Jeffrey L. Jackson et al., it is known not to have an effect on chronic tension-type headaches. The patho-

physiology of headaches which occur from temporal anchoring procedures is not known.

- Among headaches occurring after the temporal anchoring procedure, there are some cases that do not respond to analgesics but respond effectively to botulinum toxin. We think that there is a vascular factor associated with the headache. Further research and establishing clear treatment standards for this would be necessary.

3. To treat headaches of patients with temporal muscle hypertrophy, if botulinum toxin is injected, an additional slimming effect of wide head shape can be obtained.

**Tip!**

Tips for Proceeding a Cannula

- It is advisable to insert a cannula at a consistent depth (if it passes superficially, the likelihood of bumps or dimples after thread insertion increases).
- Entry point, zygomatic arch: There are not much fat between the SMAS and dermis in this area. If a cannula is inserted with a feeling of right below the subdermis rather than close to the SMAS, it proceeds smoothly at an adequate depth within the subcutaneous layer.

## 23.4   Adequate Cannula for Long-Thread Insertion (17G)

It consists of two components, internal needle and external sheath, and is approximately 15–20 cm in length.

### 23.4.1  Method of Using Inner Guide Needle (Blunt) + Sharp Outer Sheath (One Pair) (Figs. 23.9b, 23.10, and 23.11)

*Disadvantages*

- Much force is needed when it penetrates the skin.
- Sharp outer sheath gets resistance when passing through tissues. Sometimes a hair follicle gets caught at the end of the bevel.

### 23.4.2  Method of Using Inner Guide Needle (Blunt) + Blunt Outer Sheath (One Pair) and Sharp Inner Puncture Needle (Fig. 23.9a, Fig. 23.12, Fig. 23.17)

*Advantages*

- Inserting a thread into the outer sheath is convenient as the entrance of outer sheath is cut in oblique shape.

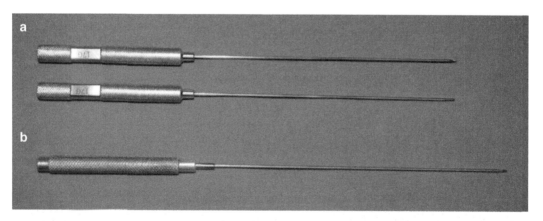

**Fig. 23.9** Tools for the fascia anchoring method – two types of cannula sets. (**a**) Two needles + one sheath method. (**b**) one needle + one sheath method

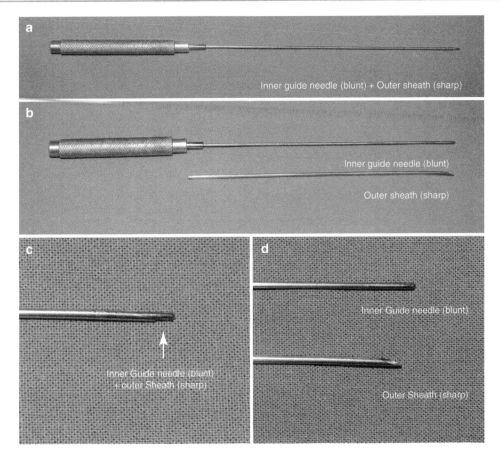

**Fig. 23.10** Tools for the fascia anchoring method – one needle + one sheath method. (**a**) Inner guide needle (blunt) combined with outer sheath (sharp). (**b**) Inner guide needle (blunt) separated from outer sheath (sharp). (**c**) (Magnification of the end part of **a**/arrow indicates end of the sheath) As the guide needle is longer than the bevel of the sheath, when it enters in the combined status, dam-ages within the tissues are minimized. Sometimes, tissues get caught at the end of the bevel. (**d**) (Magnification of the end part of **b**) As there is a bevel at the end of the sheath in the opposite direction from the handle, it is sharp. It penetrates the skin at the exit point by using the sheath with itself separated from the guide needle

## 23.5 Cutting and Finishing

Cutting is not done right after inserting threads but after pulling the procedure part more.

### 23.5.1 Finishing (Pulling)

With one hand hold both ends of the thread at the exit, and fix the skin at the cog/cone after moving the skin to the direction from the original location to the entry point using the other hand with the feeling that the cog is caught in the skin(viz., while the thread stays in the original location, push and lift the skin toward the entry point). Repeat this process twice or thrice. While this process takes place, an assistance must be pressing the anchoring point using his/her hand. If the physician pulls the thread too strongly without this, tearing of the anchoring point can happen (see Fig. 23.11m temporal fixation).

### 23.5.2 Cutting

While holding the thread, push the skin upward by approximately 4–5 mm at the exit point, and cut the thread using scissors in the other hand.

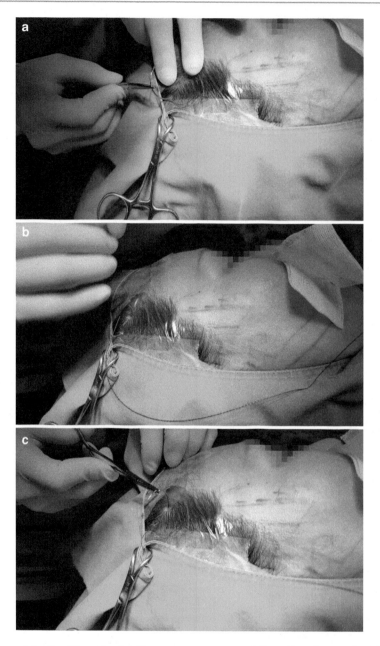

**Fig. 23.11** Temporal fixation (41 cm long) – U pattern. (**a**) To insert a long thread, firstly use a long needle to perform anchoring in the temporal area. (**b**) Insert the thread into the hole at the end of the needle. (**c**) Using the needle holder, pull out the entire needle from the entry point in the other side. (**d**) Once the entire needle passes through, separate the thread from the needle. (**e**) Pull so that each half of the thread hangs in the two entry points in a "U" shape. (**f**) Insert a long cannula at the first entry point (Fig. 23.12a blunt guide needle + sheath) and passing through the subcutaneous layer. (**g**) Penetrate and pass toward the exit (first separate the blunt guide needle out of the sheath, and insert the puncture needle in Fig. 23.12a into the sheath. Then, using the other hand, grab the for- ceps, support the exit, and come through the skin with force in the right hand) (see Fig. 23.17g–h). (**h**) If the puncture needle is separated from the sheath, only the sheath stays in between the entry point and the exit. (**i**) Insert the thread through the sheath from the entry point to the exit. (**j**) Pull and remove the sheath from the other side. (**k**) After the sheath is being removed, only the cog thread is left underneath the skin. (**l**) If the remaining half of the thread is inserted using the same method, one long thread hangs in a "U" shape. (**m**) While gently lifting the skin upward with the other hand, fix the cog on the skin. (**n**) Finally, cut the thread (press the skin upward with disinfected scissor and cut with one to two cogs out), and then gently pull the skin by snapping with the finger

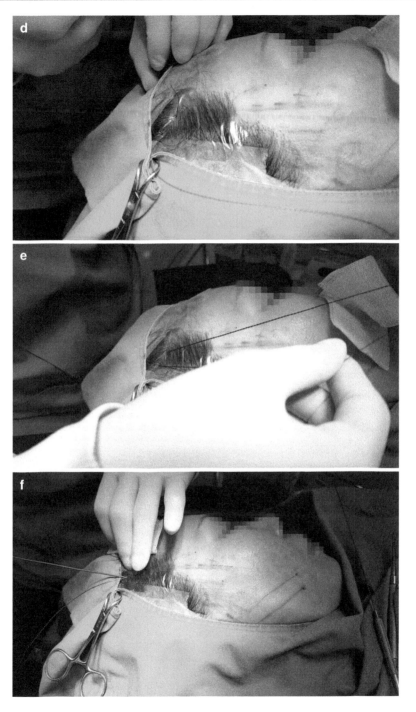

**Fig. 23.11** (continued)

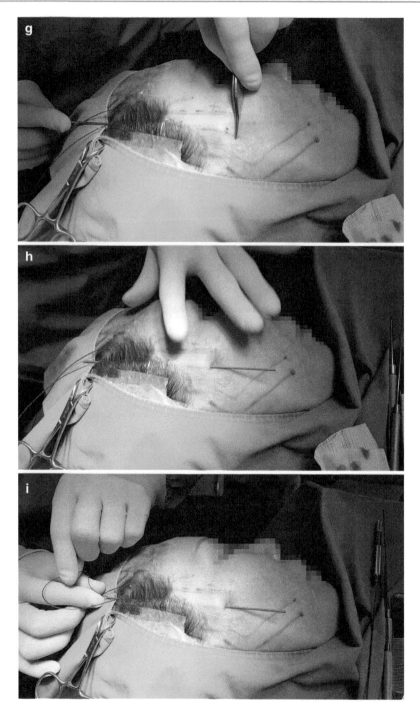

**Fig. 23.11** (continued)

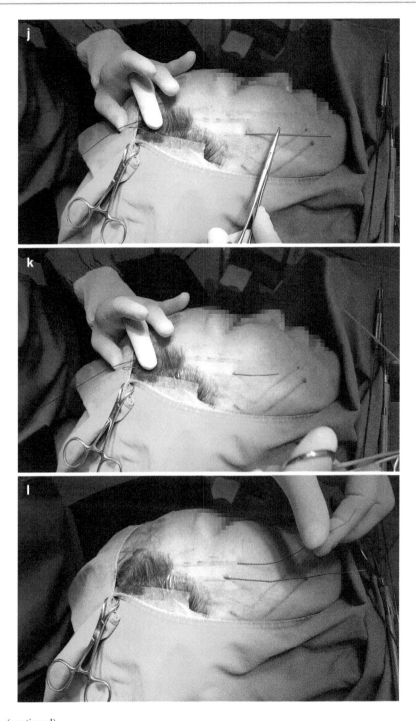

**Fig. 23.11** (continued)

**Fig. 23.11**  (continued)

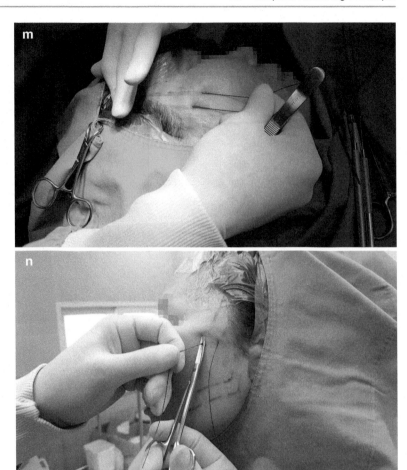

Immediately after cutting, a dimple may show at the cutting point. It can be easily resolved by gently pulling the skin downward by snapping the tissue using the thumb or index finger below the exit (see Fig. 23.11n temporal fixation).

### 23.5.3  Changes in the Skin Around the Entry Point (Dimple)

After completing the procedure, it is normal to have the skin around the entry point to be slightly folded upward.

### 23.5.4  Fine Wrinkles Around the Eyes and (Distortion of the Skin)

If there is severe skin laxity (mid to elder ages), fine wrinkles may show around the eye and tem-poral areas after procedure (Fig. 23.14). This occurs in perpendicular to the direction of the lifting direction.

In general, it disappears within few days due to gravity. Therefore, there is no need to push down the skin to restore its original form.

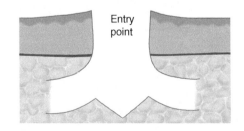

**Fig. 23.12** Tools for the fascia anchoring method – two needles + one sheath method. (**a**) Inner guide needle (blunt) combined with outer sheath. (**b**) Inner guide needle (blunt) separated from outer sheath. (**c**) (Magnification of the handle part) There is a bevel at the end of the sheath which connects to the handle. (**d**) (Magnification of the end of the opposite side) The guide needle is inserted combined with the sheath, and tissue damages are minimized when proceeding. Penetration of the skin at the exit point is performed, while the sheath and the inner puncture needle are combined

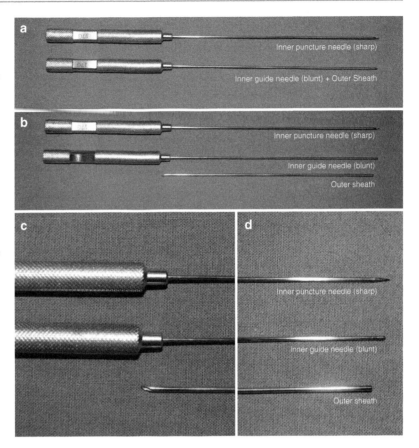

**Tip!**
How to Distinguish Procedures Which Are Within a Normal Range from Abnormal Ones
    After inserting a thread in a U shape and both ends of the thread are pulled:

- If there is no sinking in the skin near the two entry point holes, it is normal.
- If the skin near one or two entry points are concaved inward:

→ Cause (Fig. 43.9; see causes and preventions of entry point dimples).
→ Treatment: Dissection must be performed using scissors or other tools.
→ Prevention: Form a tunnel using an awl or use a temporal ring instead of a needle.

**Fig. 23.13** An example of design using the fascia anchoring method (one thread per each side)

<Design>

QT lift
long thread
41cm

x 1ea
/ each side

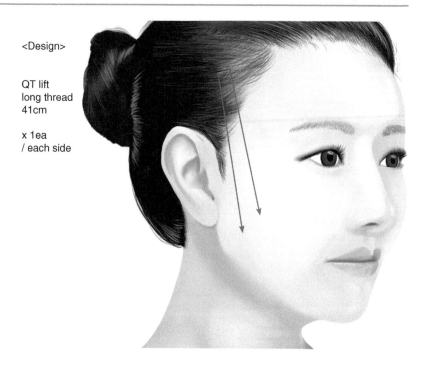

**Fig. 23.14** Areas where fine wrinkles may occur after the fascia anchoring method. If the fascia anchoring method is performed on an elderly person with thin skin, it is likely to cause barrow-shaped wrinkles in the temporal area next to the eyes. Normally it is self-healed in 2 to 3 days in general

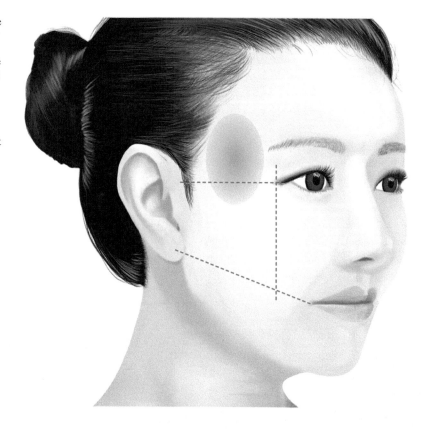

**Fig. 23.15** Photos before and after the fascia anchoring method: QT lift long thread (41 cm) × 2ea + QT lift 18 cm (L Shape Technique) × 2ea / each side

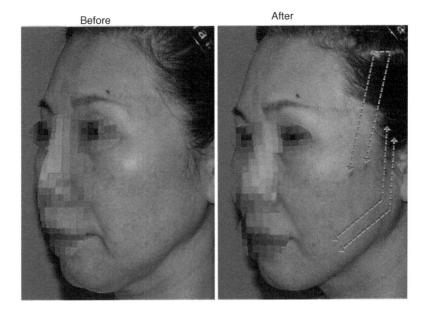

Before After

**Fig. 23.16** An example of design using the fascia anchoring method (two threads per each side)

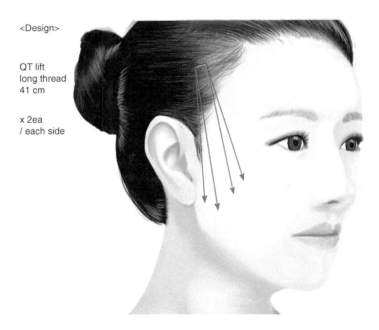

<Design>

QT lift
long thread
41 cm

x 2ea
/ each side

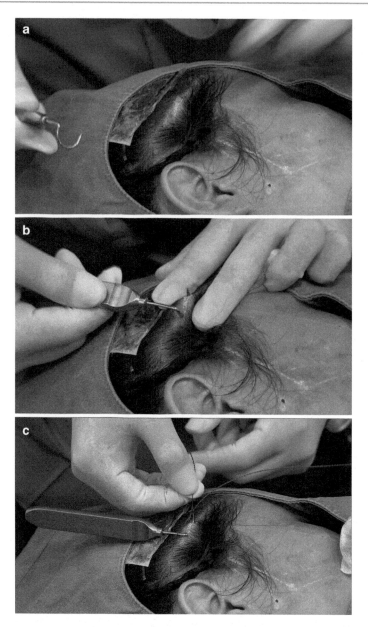

**Fig. 23.17** Temporal fixation (41 cm long) – U pattern: two threads per side using the temporal ring. (**a**) Hold the temporal ring which looks like a half ring at the end. (**b**) Insert one through one entry point first, and exit from the other entry point again after anchoring the temporal ring while it is being revolved. (**c**) Insert each thread in the two holes at the end of the ring (for a tool with two holes, the procedure time can be saved by inserting two threads at once). (**d**) Remove the temporal ring from the other side again while revolving it. (**e**) Remove the ring and pull the thread in a "U" shape so that each half of the thread hangs in the two entry points. (**f**) Insert a long cannula in the first entry point (Fig. 23.12a blunt guide needle + sheath), pass the thread at the same depth in the subcutaneous layer, and go up to the front of the exit. (**g**) Separate and remove the blunt guide needle from the sheath. (**h**) Only the sheath remains. Insert the puncture needle in Fig. 23.12a into the sheath. (**i**) Using the other hand, grab the forceps, support the exit, and prepare to pass the puncture needle from exit with force in the right hand. (**j**) If the puncture needle is separated from the sheath, only the sheath hangs in between the entry point and the exit. (**k**) Insert the thread into one entry point of the sheath, and cause it to come out of the exit. The following process is identical to **j–n** in Fig. 23.11

**Fig. 23.17** (continued)

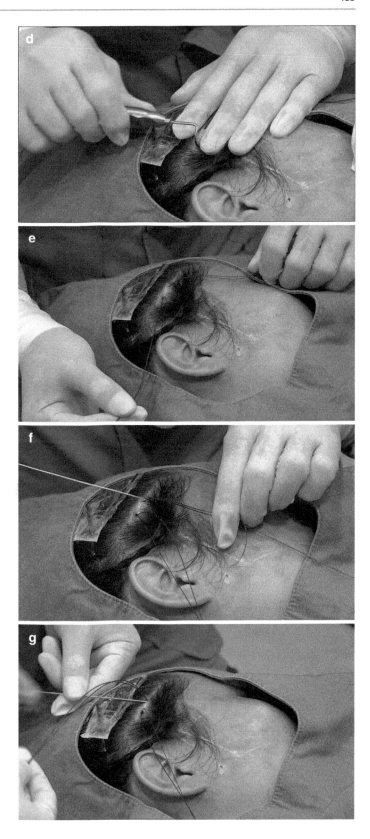

**Fig. 23.17** (continued)

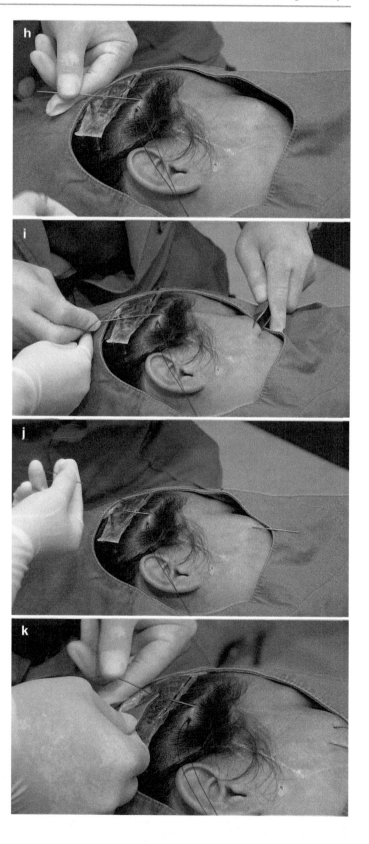

**Fig. 23.18** Temporal
fixation (41 cm
long) – U pattern: two
lines per side using a
temporal ring. (**a**) QT
lift 41 cm × 4 ea. (**b**) QT
lift 41 cm × 4ea (face
lifting), QT lift
41 cm × 2ea (submental
lifting)

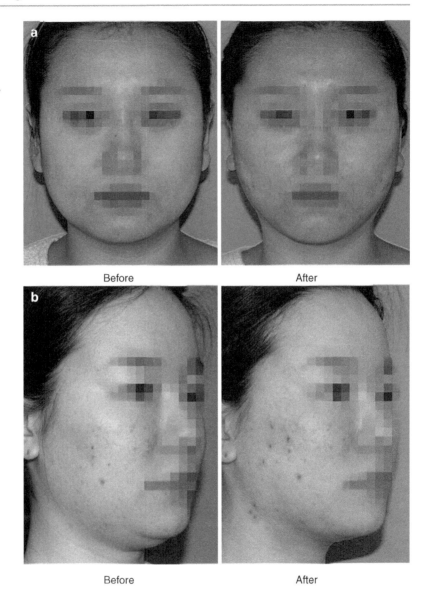

Before            After

Before            After

## 24.1 Mechanisms (Concept)

We dealt with bi-directional cog threads in the previous chapter. In this chapter, we introduce bi-directional threads with cones rather than cogs. This method is convenient for performing without a cannula as the two ends of the thread are connected to a needle. This type of thread is called as a thread with a bi-directional needle. Silhouette Soft® is a representative one.

Silhouette Soft® threads consist of poly-L-lactic acid (PLLA) ingredient. This ingredient decomposes and absorbs in the body. This is one of absorbable threads.

### 24.1.1 Effect of Silhouette Soft®

1. Its cones bind well with the subcutaneous tissues immediately after the procedure and display immediate lifting effects.
2. As time passes, new collagen is formed around the cones and the thread. It provides additional elasticity by supporting nearby soft tissues.

### 24.1.2 Exclusive Advantages of Silhouette Soft®

Instead of cogs, there are cones, which are not fixed and capable of moving in the space between knots (approximately 0.5–0.8 mm), thereby

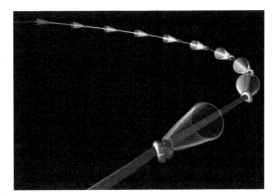

**Fig. 24.1** Several knots and cones exist in both directions (bi-directional). (Source: Silhouette Soft®/SINCLAIR), https://www.sinclairpharma.com/silhouette-soft

almost no dimple is created from hanging of cogs (Fig. 24.1). This is a new lifting in a concept of fat redispositioning.

## 24.2 Characteristics

### 24.2.1 Structure

It has a structure of connecting a bi-directional thread with cones and needles in both ends of the thread. Depending on the number of cones, there are three types of threads (8 cones, 12 cones, and 16 cones). For each type of the thread, the same number of cones is spread in half in each side. The two ends of the thread are connected to a needle of 12 cm in length and 23G in thickness (Fig. 24.2).

© Springer Nature Singapore Pte Ltd. 2019
B. Kim et al., *The Art and Science of Thread Lifting*, https://doi.org/10.1007/978-981-13-0614-3_24

There is a knot between the cones. Namely, cones drive freely between the knots. The space between the knots is 0.5 cm in case of 8 cones and 0.8 cm in case of 12 cones and 16 cones. The length of the space between the knots at the center of the thread where a cone does not exist is 2 cm.

## 24.2.2 Ingredients

The thread is composed of poly-L-lactic acid (PLLA) ingredient. Cones consisted of poly-L-lactic acid (82%) and glycolic polymer (18%). These ingredients decompose and are absorbed. PLLA is absorbed within 30 months.

**Table 24.1** Composition of bi-directional needle + bi-directional cones (Silhouette Soft®)

| Product | Soft 8 cones | Soft 12 cones | Soft 16 cones |
|---|---|---|---|
| USP designation | | 3.0 | |
| Length | 30 cm | 27.5 cm | 26.8 cm |
| Number of cones | 8 | 12 | 16 |
| Direction of the cones | Bi-directional | | |
| Space between cones | 5 mm | 8 mm | 8 mm |
| Material | | PLA | |
| Needle | 2 needles (23G) of 12 cm each | | |

## 24.2.3 Preparations for the Procedure

Preparations are simple compared to lifting with other threads. It is similar to thread lifting using disposable cannulas. Simple configuration and standardized techniques allow consistent procedures anywhere in the world.

- Design rule: Mandatory item as distance measurement is essential for designing
- Anesthetic solution: Dental lidocaine (lidocaine 1% with epinephrine 1:100,000)
- 18G needle: entry point puncture

## 24.3 Method of the Procedure

### 24.3.1 Designing

1. Exit
   In designing, the length from an entry point to an exit must be made with extra room (viz., it should not be shorter than the minimum required distance) (see Fig. 24.3). The minimum required distance is longer than the distance between the center of thread and the outermost knot. When designing, we must consider the movement of the soft tissue by lifting. If there is severe sagging, it can be designed 1 cm longer

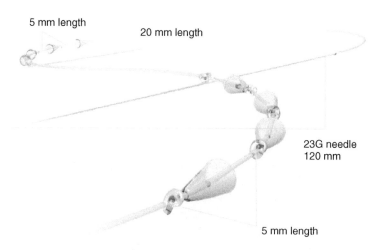

**Fig. 24.2** Example of bi-directional needle + bi-directional cones. (Source: Silhouette Soft®/SINCLAIR), https://www.sinclairpharma.com/silhouette-soft

5 mm length

20 mm length

23G needle 120 mm

5 mm length

than the minimum required distance shown in the table below for more traction.

In case of asymmetry, it is advisable to make an exit point 0.5–1 cm farther than usual at the time of designing (if you make a traction more than the standard, a knot or cone can tag along through the exit).

2. Route of the thread (vector)

It is advisable that beginners should avoid the curve vector in designing passage in a "U" pattern.

3. Entry point
4. Summary of draping and hairline

## 24.3.2  Anesthesia

- Anesthetic solution: Dental lidocaine (lidocaine 1% with epinephrine 1:100,000)
- Area: entry point and exit are enough (Fig. 24.4).

**Table 24.2**  Design length for each number of cones (minimum required distance)

| Minimum required distance between the entry point and each exit point for all patterns | |
| --- | --- |
| 8 cones suture | 6 cm |
| 12 cones suture | 9 cm |
| 16 cones suture | 11 cm |

There is no need to anesthetize the entire route.

If additional anesthesia is necessary in areas other than the entry point and the exit:

- Patients who are largely worried about pain.
- When patients claim pain during the procedure.
- If the exit is near to the mouth (as the subcutaneous tissues near the mouth are dense, needles do not pass through easily, thereby more pain occurs and likelihood of bleeding increases). A dimple is easily formed at this area. But cones of Silhouette Soft® are not fixed and they can move between knots. Therefore, no dimple occurs even when procedures are done in this area (see Fig. 23.6).

## 24.3.3  Entry point (Fig. 24.5)

1. Entry point puncture tool

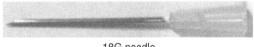

18G needle

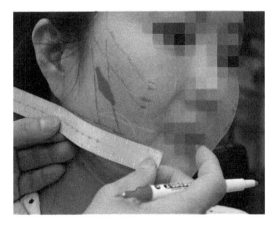

**Fig. 24.3**  Prior to performing procedure of bi-directional needle + bi-directional cones (Silhouette soft®), the minimum required distance between the entry point to the exit must be kept (©Medbook Co., Ltd. All rights reserved)

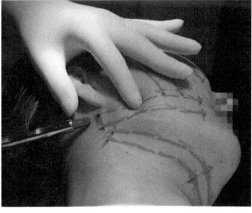

**Fig. 24.4**  Procedures of bi-directional needle + bi-directional cones (Silhouette Soft®) – anesthesia with dental lidocaine (©Medbook Co., Ltd. All rights reserved)

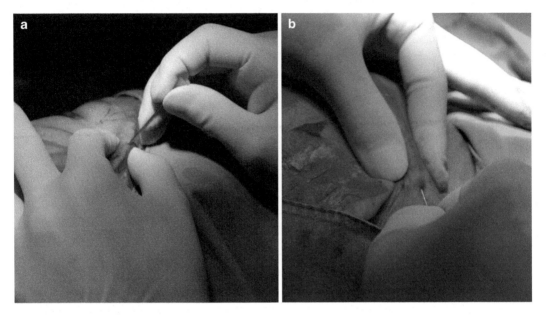

**Fig. 24.5** Procedures of bi-directional needle + bi-directional cones (Silhouette soft®) – entry point. (**a**) Making an entry point using a 18G needle. (**b**) Showing of a Silhouette Soft® needle being inserted through an entry point

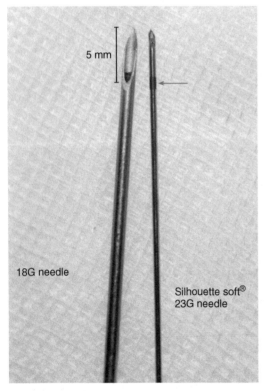

**Fig. 24.6** Procedures of bi-directional needle + bi-directional cones (Silhouette Soft®) – bevel of 18G needle, black line at the end of the 23G Silhouette Soft® needle

2. Puncture technique

   In puncturing a hole with a 18G needle, pinch the skin with the other hand, insert the needle perpendicularly with a slight stir (revolving), and dissect the subcutaneous tissues from the dermis below the entry point. In that way, dimples can be prevented.

   Enter up to the depth of approximately 5 mm. This depth is identical to the length of the 18 G needle bevel (Fig. 24.6).

3. Insertion of 23G Silhouette Soft® needle through an entry point

   Enter perpendicularly up to the depth of 5 mm (Fig. 24.7). The black line at the end of the needle is the 5 mm mark line (Fig. 24.6).

**Summary**

Responding to Bleeding at the Time of Anchoring: Silhouette Soft® U Technique

1. While passing an 18G needle (puncture needle) at an entry point
   – If blood is on the connection area of the needle and plastic (Fig. 24.8), continue to proceed.

- If blood comes out continuously in the connection area (Fig. 24.8) of the needle and the plastic, remove and perform hemostasis. Then, perform the procedure through a new entry point.
2. After a Silhouette Soft® needle (23G) passes through and an 18G needle is removed, if bleeding occurs at the entry point and does not stop
   - If the thread has passed the anchoring point, cut the very center of the thread, remove it, and perform hemostasis. In this case, the Silhouette Soft® cannot be reused (if the Silhouette Soft® needle [23 g] has passed entirely, the needle cannot be pulled back. The connecting area of the needle and the thread must be cut and removed).
   - If bleeding occurs after the Silhouette Soft® needle (23G) passes the anchoring point partially, pull back the needle and perform hemostasis.

Therefore, in anchoring:

1. Check how much blood got on the connecting part of the needle and the plastic.
2. If you check the bleeding when only a portion of the Silhouette Soft® needle passes the anchoring point, there is no need for throwing out Silhouette Soft® unnecessarily.

**Fig. 24.7** Procedures of bi-directional needle + bi-directional cones (Silhouette Soft®) – a cross section of inserted 23G Silhouette Soft® needle. (Published with kind permission of © Kwan- Hyun Youn 2018. All rights reserved)

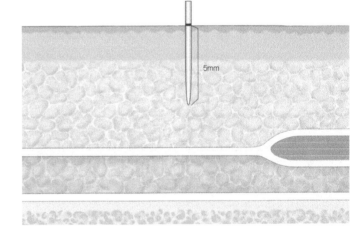

5mm

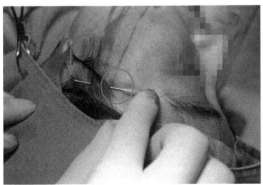
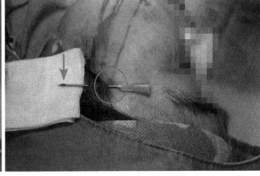

**Fig. 24.8** Needle with blood on. Although little blood got on at the end of the needle, as the connecting part of the needle and the plastic does not show any blood on, continue to proceed with the procedure. Even if there is little blood that got on the connecting part of the needle and the plastic, it is OK to proceed with the procedure. However, if there is any blood coming out from the connecting part of the needle and the plastic, stop the procedure and perform hemostasis after removing

### 24.3.4 Insertion (Fig. 24.9)

1. Method of holding a needle
   - Hold on to the shortest as possible closely to the entry point (if the needle is held long, it bends well during insertion).
   - Hold with the thumb and the index finger.

- In the temporal muscle (TM) hypertrophy/trigonocephaly, the needle must be held closely to the nail to insert horizontally. In such case, if the needle is held by the middle of the distal phalanx (Fig. 24.10), the needle will insert more deeply as it proceeds.

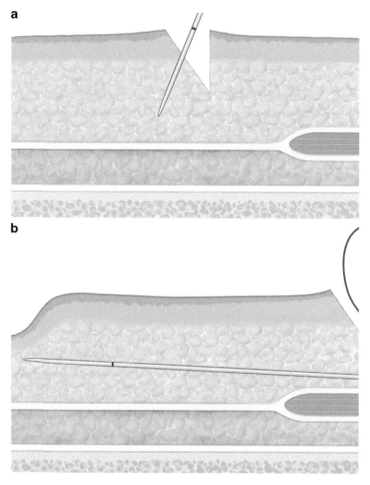

**Fig. 24.9** Cross section of inserting the bi-directional needle + bi-directional cones (Silhouette Soft®). (**a**) Insert the end of the needle in one side of the Silhouette Soft® perpendicularly into the subcutaneous tissues. Insert up to the point that the black line at the end of the needle touches the skin at the entry point so that the depth is 5 mm. (**b**) To maintain the needle horizontally, proceed toward the exit at a consistent depth in the subcutaneous tissues. Then, the needle comes out puncturing the exit. (Published with kind permission of © Kwan- Hyun Youn 2018. All rights reserved). (**c**) Pull the needle gently to outside (retract) and cause cones to enter the subcutaneous tissues gently along the thread. After the last cone is inserted and half of the entire thread is inserted, stop retraction. (**d**) Insert the remaining side of the needle using the same method. After inserting the end of the needle perpendicularly into the subcutaneous tissues, change the direction and proceed toward the exit horizontally. (**e**) The needle punctures the exit and comes out. Thereafter, gently pull the needle to outside and insert the remaining cones gently into the subcutaneous tissues. (Published with kind permission of © Kwan-Hyun Youn 2018. All rights reserved). (**f, g**) Once the entire thread and cones are inserted into the subcutaneous tissues, cut the connecting part of the needle and the thread first. The thread must remain long in both exits. While holding one side of the thread with one hand, fix the cones, pushing up the skin toward the desired direction using the other hand (traction). (Published with kind permission of © Kwan- Hyun Youn 2018. All rights reserved)

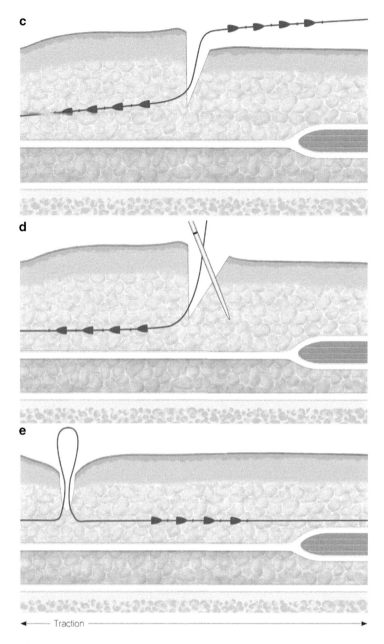

**Fig. 24.9** (continued)

**Fig. 24.9** (continued)

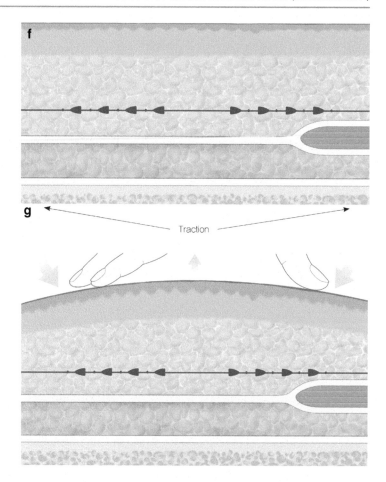

**Summary**
Method of Inserting a Needle at a Constant Depth Using Pinch Technique (Fig. 24.11)

- Finger pinch
  - Point pinch: useful in making an entry point
  - Block pinch: after inserting into an entry point and until entering up to about the first 1/3 of the insertion route
- V pinch
  - When passing the middle part of insertion route
  - Especially useful in the submental area

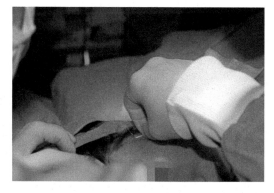

**Fig. 24.10** Method of inserting a needle in the temporal muscle (TM) hypertrophy/trigonocephaly. In holding a needle, use the middle of the distal phalanx of the thumb and the index finger in general. However, in the temporal muscle (TM) hypertrophy/trigonocephaly, horizontal insertion can be done at a constant depth only if the needle is held by the end of the phalanx closely to the nails as shown above (©Medbook Co., Ltd. All rights reserved)

- Press
  - When passing the last 1/3 of insertion route.
  - Press the skin right on the insertion route with the distal phalanges of the second, third, and fourth fingers.
  - Useful when passing the curvy area of the cheek or dense fibrotic area.
  - When passing the curve of the cheek, it is easier to pass by pressing on the skin of the end of the needle. If the needle is bent, it would be more convenient to pass.

**Summary**
Method of Checking the Depth After Inserting a Needle

- This is a process of checking whether a needle is inserted at a consistent depth in the subcutaneous fat from the entry point to the exit point.
- When a needle penetrates through the exit, instead of pulling it out straight, hold both ends of the needle with two hands and bend the needle toward the top of the skin (Fig. 24.12).
  - Check if the needle is uniformly inserted within the subcutaneous fat.
- If the thickness of the lifted tissue through a bent needle is not uniform, it is advisable to withdraw the needle and proceed again. If cones are inserted at inconsistent depth, traction does not work well or skin folds may occur; therefore cautions must be taken.
  - Solution: If a needle is inserted by proceeding straight slowly using suitable technique for each area, it can be performed at a consistent depth.

**Summary**
Cause and Prevention of Breakage of a Thread When It Passes Through

1. Cause of breakage while a thread passes through
   Excessive pulling of thread
2. Prevention (technique)
   The force of the hand used in pulling a needle must be controlled. It is also important to push the skin with opposite hand so that the cones enter into the tissues easily without being trapped.
   - Hand which pulls the needle
     - Hold the needle as close as possible to the exit point while pulling.
     - If holding is done far away from the exit point, as much force is hung, there is a risk of the thread being cut.
   - Opposite hand
     Push the skin in the opposite direction.
     - When the first cone enters into the entry point
     - When more than half of the cones are inserted

**Summary**
Method of Gentle Retraction Without Having the Thread Cut While It Passes Through (Fig. 24.13)

1. First stage
   When the first cone passes through the entry point
2. Second stage
   When the first cone passes in the middle of insertion route (when the cone in the middle part of the thread passes the entry point)
3. Third stage
   When the last cone passes through the entry point

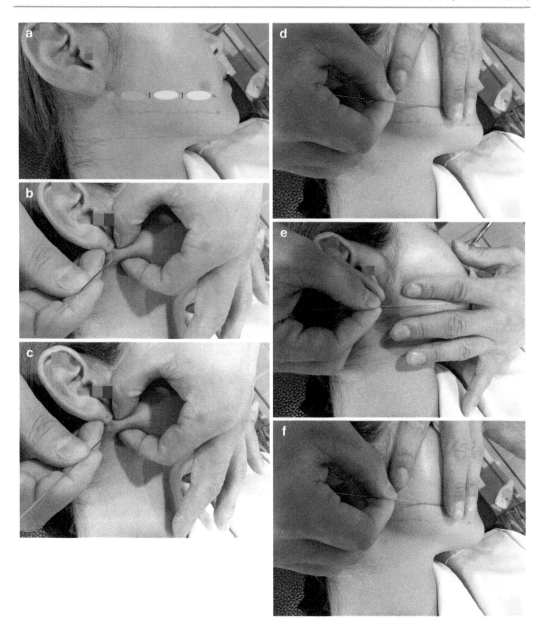

**Fig. 24.11** Procedure of Silhouette Soft® – inserting needle using various pinch techniques for each area. (**a**) This shows the design for lower face lifting technique using U pattern (see Fig. 24.19). Each from the left shows the entry point (red), proximal 1/3 (blue), middle 1/3 (green), and distal 1/3 (apricot). (**b**) Point pinch (hard): in making an entry point using a puncturing needle, hold the skin around the entry point with the tip of the fingers. To avoid injury of blood vessels and muscles, skin tissues must be pulled upward requiring a strong grip. (**c**) Point pinch (soft): when Silhouette Soft® needle enters through an entry point, grip gently with the tip of the fingers. If pinching too strongly, as the entry point cannot open properly, likelihood of dimple increases. Accordingly, pinch gently so that the entry point shows slightly. (**d**) Block pinch: after inserting into the entry point and passing the proximal 1/3, grip widely with fingers to insert a needle at a constant depth within the subcutaneous fat. (**e**) V pinch: the subcutaneous fat in the middle 1/3 is very soft. Passing this area can be easily performed by pinching in a "V" shape using the second and the third fingers. (**f**) Press: the subcutaneous fat in the distal 1/3 is very dense. Inserting a needle while slightly pressing the tissues is useful for passing at a consistent depth within a dense layer

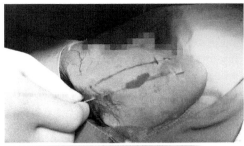

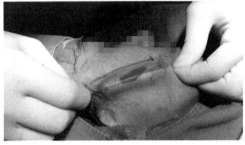

**Fig. 24.12** Procedure of Silhouette Soft® – checking an insertion depth (©Medbook Co., Ltd. All rights reserved)

**Summary**
How to Solve When the Last Cone Does Not Enter into Entry Point (Fig. 24.14)

1. Cause
   • When the last cone is not located perpendicularly in front of the entry point and lies in a horizontal position against the skin, the cone is likely to fail to enter into the entry point.
2. Solution
   • Make the cone in the horizontal position lying against the skin place in a vertical position (viz., place the tip of the isosceles triangle of the cone to face the entry point perpendicularly).
   • An assistant pulls the thread lightly with a forceps, placing the cone vertically like in Fig. 24.14b. Then, the cone enters easily by pulling.

**Vertical position**     **Horizontal position**

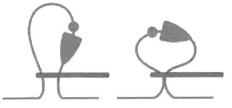

**Prevention**
• Make the length between the last cone and the center of entire thread sufficient for the cone to be positioned vertically in front of the entry point.

### 24.3.5 Cutting and Finishing (Traction, Pulling Threads)

• It is advisable to cut out a needle right after insertion (viz., perform prior to traction).
• Role of assistance in performing traction.
  – In a U pattern technique, pressing the entry point prevents the thread from coming down at the anchoring point while a physician performs traction.
• Traction.
  – Usually the thread is pulled by a physician's fingers.
  – If the thread is not long enough to be pulled, it can be pulled using a needle holder.
  – Push the skin on the last cone (bottom cone) upward so that the skin is lifted and fixed to the next cone. Once pushing the top cone is done, repeat from the bottom cone to the top cone again (some groups prefer the method of moving from the top to the bottom).
  – Repeat until the last knot becomes close to the exit.
  – Feeling click sounds brings about a good outcome.

**Summary**
Importance of Traction

We previously mentioned that authors believe that designing process is the one which decisively influences the treatment outcome among all the process of thread lifting procedure. See Part 5-1, "Designing and Choice of Patients."

During thread lifting training, designing of both sides is done by the trainer (the author). Thereafter, the author inserts the threads on the right side, and the trainee performs procedures on the other side.

There is not much difference in the results from the right side and the left side. However, in case of Silhouette Soft® training, there is some difference in the results.

Differences in traction can result in the difference of outcome.

Many cases of differences in the two sides are experienced in the results of lifting after the traction process. Through a proper "traction" process, good result can be obtained and side effects like folding of the skin can be reduced.

**Fig. 24.13** Procedure of Silhouette Soft® – gentle retraction of the thread after needle insertion. (**a**) When the first cone enters into the entry point – push the skin slightly, giving a snap with one finger from the right in front or back of the entry point toward the opposite direction of insertion route. Using the other hand, hold the connecting part of the needle and thread (viz., the closest location to the exit) and gently pull. In regard to the other hand, there is no need to give a snap like the hand touching the skin. (Published with kind permission of © Kwan-Hyun Youn 2018. All rights reserved). (**b**) When the half of cones are inserted into the subcutaneous tissue – using one or two fingers, push the skin slightly from the right on the skin area where the first cone passes (approximately the middle of the route from the entry point to the exit) toward the opposite direction of insertion route. Using the other hand, hold the connecting part of the needle and thread and then gently pull. (Published with kind permission of © Kwan- Hyun Youn 2018. All rights reserved)

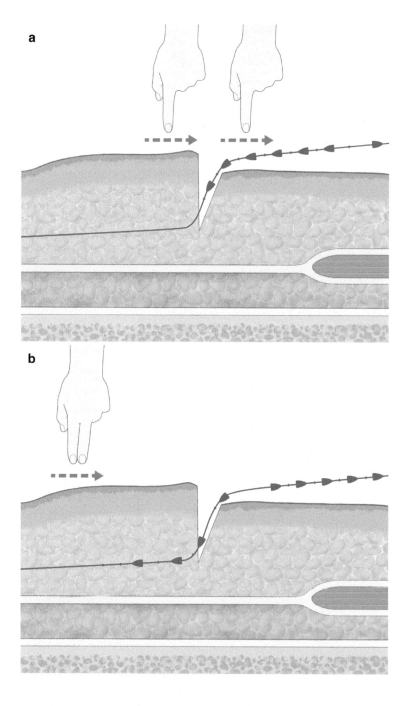

**Fig. 24.14**
Procedure of
Silhouette
Soft® – handling of
the last cone at the
entry point (**a**) The
last cone is not
located perpendicu-
larly in front of the
entry point and lies
in a horizontal
position against the
skin. (**b**) Make the
cone place in a
vertical position
using a forcep. (**c**)
Pull the thread and
release a forcep. (**d**)
The cone is inserted
correctly

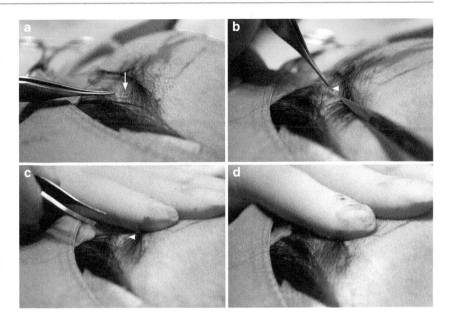

**Fig. 24.15**
Procedure of
Silhouette
Soft® – cutting
and finishing.
(**a**) Put a sterilized
scissors closely to
the exit point
where the thread
remains. (**b**) Using
a sterilized
scissors, push up
the skin and cut
closely to the last
knot. (**c**) Thread is
cut and buried
(©Medbook Co.,
Ltd. All rights
reserved)

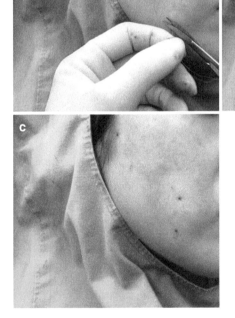

**Cutting** (Fig. 24.15)

- A thread is not to be pulled during cutting process, but the thread is to be cut while pushing
  the skin using curved scissors.
- If the exit and the last knot are too close and
  the knot should be removed, it is advisable to
  remove the last knot and the last cone

together. If the knot is removed only, the
cone next to it cannot play its role.
Furthermore, as the cone breaks away from
the thread, it can be hung in the dermis at the
exit point.

- In some cases, the end of the thread located
  around the mouth corner pokes the skin in

**Fig. 24.16** Basic technique of Silhouette Soft® – straight pattern (©Medbook Co., Ltd. All rights reserved)

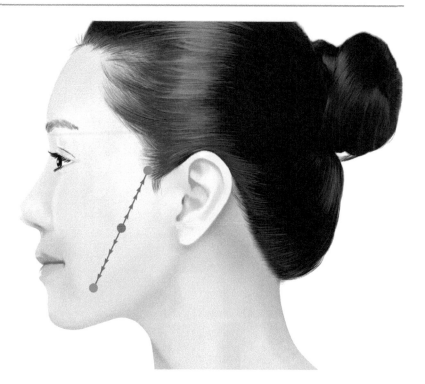

facial expression; the following cautions must be taken:

1. If the last knot is distant from the exit, it is advisable to cut after pushing the skin up to the very front of the last knot.
2. Rather than cutting in an oblique angle to the thread, cutting must be done perpendicularly, thereby reducing damage to the tissue even if it pokes the skin during facial expressions.

## 24.4 Various Techniques

### 24.4.1 Basic Technique 1: Straight Technique

1. Design (Fig. 24.16)
   This is a useful technique for patient who has partially sagged jowl rather than patient who has much volume in cheek fat.
   - Exit in the bottom: The last cone (bottom) should be fixed in the jowl.
   - Exit in the top: The last cone (top) should be fixed around the hairline.
   - Entry point: In the middle of the two exit points.

2. Anesthesia – dental lidocaine
   - Anesthetize one entry point and two exit points.
3. Cutting and traction
   - Thread in the back: Pull the thread upward first and then manipulate the thread in the front (supporting/fixing role).
   - Thread in the front: While holding the thread with one hand, by pushing the skin upward with the other hand, cause the cone in one compartment above the original cone to hang.

### 24.4.2 Basic Technique 2: Angle Technique

1. Designing (Fig. 24.17)
   - Entry point: approximately 1FB inside from the mandibular angle or right behind
   - Insertion route of lower half of the thread: If it is too close to the mandibular line, it improves only the jawline, not the marionette line. If it is located on the extension line from oral commissure to the tragus, the level is too high. It is advisable that the exit point in the bottom (exit point in

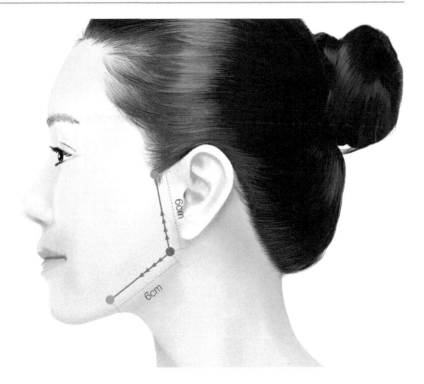

lower half of the thread) is located in the middle of above two routes. When the angle between each half of the thread is greater than the angle between the mandibular body and ramus, it can bring a better result.

2. Anesthesia – dental lidocaine
   - Anesthetize one entry point and two exits.
3. Entry point – caution/location
   - This is a technique in which a dimple frequently occurs at the entry point after the procedure.
   - If the entry point is located inside from the mandibular angle, it is likely to be exposed.
   - Prior to the procedure, puncture a hole at an entry point slightly larger than other areas using a needle or an awl.
4. Cutting and traction
   - Thread in the back (upper half of the thread): It plays a supporting or fixing role.
   - Thread in the front (lower half of the thread): While holding the thread with one hand, push the skin to the entry point with the other hand so that the skin is lifted and fixed to the next cone.

### 24.4.3 Basic Technique 3: U Technique

1. Designing (Fig. 24.18)
   One thread is used, but it has a similar effect with using two cog threads in this technique. Twelve cones and 16 cones are mainly used.
   - Entry point: Set above the hairline but between the lateral canthus level and zygomatic arch level.
   - Exit points are generally set toward the marionette line or jowl. If you want to improve the nasolabial fold, set two exits toward the nasolabial folds. .
2. Anesthesia – dental lidocaine
   - Anesthetize two entry points and two exits.
   - Anesthetize the space between the two entry points.
3. Entry point – cautions/location
   - When designing entry points, check the sentinel vein with the naked eye, and check the STA pulse by palpation to avoid vessel injury.
4. Insertion
   - For beginners, U pattern would be difficult when passing a curve in zygomatic arch. Therefore, it is advisable to avoid designing

**Fig. 24.18** Basic
technique of Silhouette
Soft® – U pattern
(©Medbook Co., Ltd.
All rights reserved)

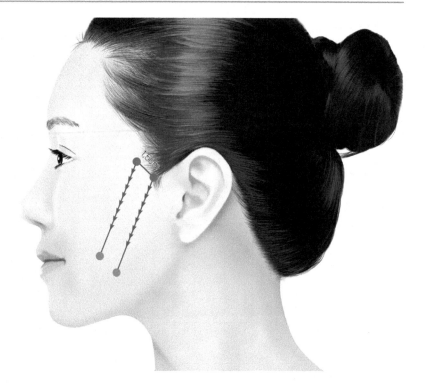

on the curvy surface if possible. Especially, as the curves of the zygomatic arch are more severe in Asians, cautions must be taken.

5. Cutting and traction
   - The directions of cones on both sides of the thread are identical.
   - Traction can be done with holding both sides of the thread or each half of the thread separately.
   - Push the skin on the last cone (bottom cone) upward so that the skin is lifted and fixed to the next cone. Some expert groups prefer the method of moving from the top to the bottom.

horizontally for passing. When it comes out through the opposite entry point, the result depends on the direction of the bevel.
   - If the bevel of the needle passes facing upward: Useful to come out through the opposite entry point.
   - If the bevel of the needle passes facing downward: It comes out puncturing new entry point after passing 3–4 mm further from the desired entry point.

**Summary**
Tips for Passing an 18G Needle (Puncture Needle) at Entry Point

1. Tips for passing needles easily through two entry points
   - When puncturing a hole using an 18G needle, after pinching the skin with the other hand, insert the needle perpendicularly, and then make it lie

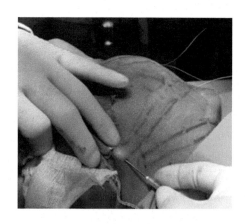

2. Tips for passing the needle easily through two entry points
   - When the bevel of the 18G needle passes facing downward around the hairline, it is likely to anchor too deep, and the risk of STA damage increases from the author's experience. If the bevel of the needle passes facing upward, the risk of bleeding can be reduced.

   → Therefore, when anchoring with 18G in U technique, it is advisable to pass a needle with the bevel facing upward.

### 24.4.4 Post-mandibular Anchoring (PMA) Technique

1. Designing (post-mandibular anchoring using U technique) (see Fig. 24.19):

- In performing a marionette line lifting using L technique or U technique, it is necessary to check prior to the procedure through simulation, whether lifting works well or not.
- In sagging of the jowl or the marionette line, two vectors (see Fig. 24.20) should be considered. They are a vector facing upward (from the mandibular body through the zygomatic bone to the temple) and a vector facing backward (from the mentalis muscle to the mandibular angle).
- When the angle between the mandibular body and the horizontal line is high, as the two vectors explained above work similarly, the procedure which pulls toward the back of the ear can make a sufficient lifting effect. Therefore, if the lifting for jowl is performed only by this technique, a greater angle displays a better effect than a smaller angle (Fig. 24.21).

**Fig. 24.19** Applied technique of the Silhouette Soft® – PMA technique (©Medbook Co., Ltd. All rights reserved)

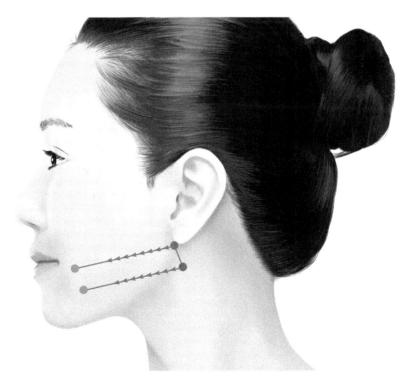

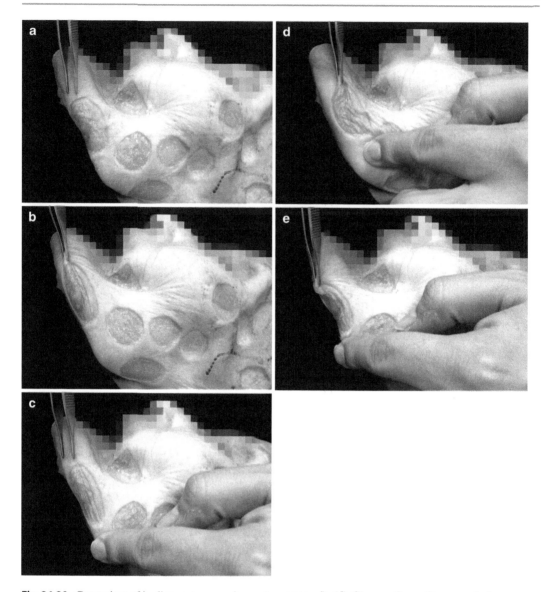

**Fig. 24.20** Comparison of jawline vectors – supine position. (**a**) Cadaver of the supine position (intact state not pulled). (**b**) Change after pulling anteriorly – vector toward the mentalis muscle. (**c**) Change after pulling posteriorly – vector toward the mandibular angle. (Published with kind permission of © Wonsug Jung 2018. All rights reserved). (**d**) Change after pulling superiorly – vector toward the zygomatic arch (temple). (**e**) Change after pulling inferiorly – vector toward the submental area. (Published with kind permission of © Wonsug Jung 2018. All rights reserved)

**Summary**

Factors Which Affect the Outcome of the PMA Technique

- When the effect is good
  - When the angle between the mandibular body and the horizontal line is high (30° or above)

- When the effect is poor
  - When the angle between the mandibular body and the horizontal line is low (below 20°)
  - Patients with a square jaw (–> this can make the square jaw to be more prominent)

**Fig. 24.21** Factors which affect the outcome of the PMA technique

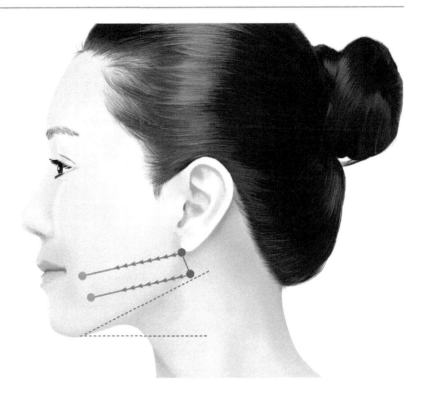

2. Anesthesia – dental lidocaine
   - Anesthetize two entry points and two exits.
   - Anesthetize the space between the two entry points.
3. Entry point – cautions/location
   - It is advisable to set the entry point right behind the mandible angle, below the ear.
4. Insertion
   - When a needle passes from the entry point to the exit, the density of the fat tissues is various depending on each area. It is more useful to insert thread using pinch techniques (see various pinch techniques for each area in Fig. 24.22).
5. Cutting and traction
   - It is the same as basic U technique.

## 24.4.5  Various Combinations Using Two Threads

> **Tip!**
> Tips for Overcoming Disadvantages of the Crisscross Technique and Making Favorable Effects

- A crossing point shall not be the bulging area in the cheekbone (the space between the cheekbone and the ear).
- Attempting to perform traction simultaneously after inserting two threads, a desired outcome is not obtained well. After performing insertion and traction for one thread, it would be better to insert the second one and then perform traction.
- It is advisable to have the crossing point near the entry point. This is because the crisscross point can act as a secondary fixing point following the entry point, and function of the fixing point can be enhanced. If this is utilized well, we can expect a good result.
- If the temples are sunk, we can expect a good volumizing effect by making a crossing point in this area (however, in case of sunken cheeks, the inner vector, rather than the downward vector, reacts together (or reacts more), and it is difficult to expect a smooth volumization like fillers).

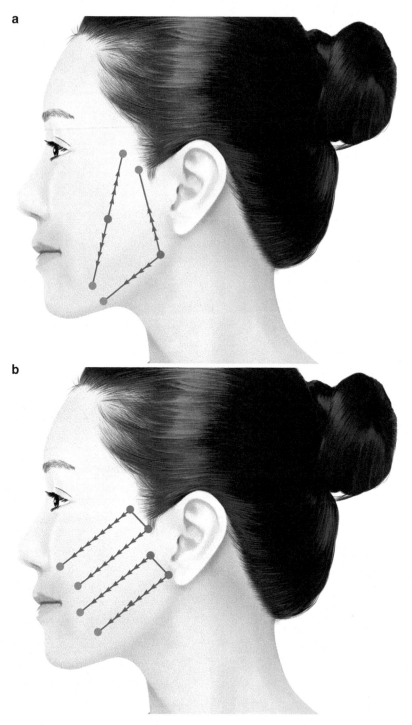

**Fig. 24.22** Applied techniques of the Silhouette Soft® – various combinations. (**a**) Straight + angle technique. (**b**) Method of using two U techniques. (**c**) Crisscross technique. (**d**) Straight + angle technique

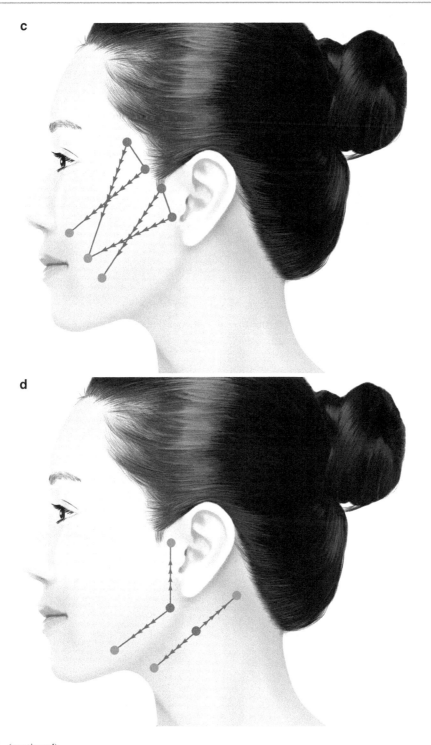

**Fig. 24.22** (continued)

**Summary**

Cautions in the Crisscross Technique

It can provide volumizing effects if done on sunken areas, but there are various considerations.

- First of all, it is difficult to pass (especially in case of thick cog thread).
- It is also difficult to insert additional thread later even if a small thread is selected.
- In case of those who have developed zygomatic arch, it is advisable not to have the crossing part in the zygomatic arch. The zygomatic arch may appear to be more bulging.
- When performed on the sunken cheek, the shape might become strange due to tangling of threads and tissues. Cautions must be taken.
- The skin does not move much in the process of cutting and pulling the thread in crisscross technique case.
- The crossing point shall not be on the zygomatic arch. It must be more to the side of the zygomatic arch (the space between the zygomatic bone and the ear).

**Tip!**

Tips for solving wide dents of the skin after the criss-cross technique

After putting the other hand inside the mouth and mold while pushing the skin with the finger, the tangled cones detangle well.

## 24.4.6 Eyebrow Lifting (Fig. 24.23)

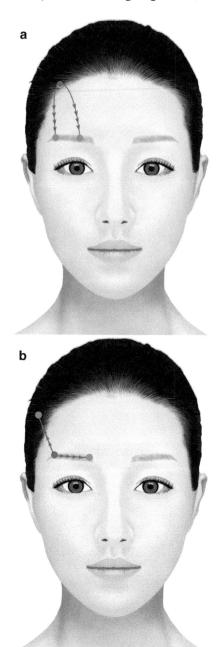

**Fig. 24.23** Applied techniques of the Silhouette Soft® – forehead lifting (**a**) U technique (**b**) Angle technique (©Medbook Co., Ltd. All rights reserved)

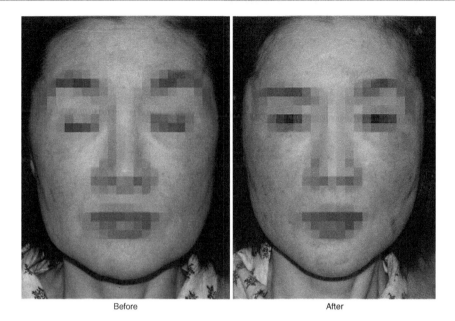

Before                    After

**Fig. 24.24** Combined procedure of the Silhouette Soft® and bi-directional cog thread – photos before and after the procedure. Silhouette Soft® 8 cone×4 ea. + QT lift 41 cm × 4 ea (©Medbook Co., Ltd. All rights reserved)

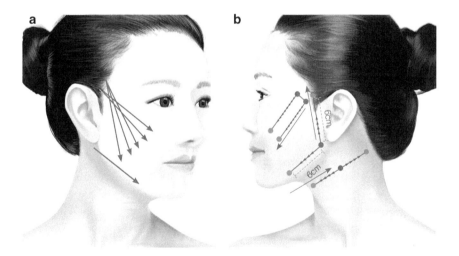

**Fig. 24.25** Difference in the directions of thread insertions. (**a**) Traditional thread. (**b**) Silhouette Soft® (©Medbook Co., Ltd. All rights reserved)

## 24.5 Useful Tips

**Summary**
Tips for the Silhouette Soft® Technique: Position of the Procedure

As other threads have similar progression vectors, it is convenient to perform the procedure by sitting at the upper side of the patient. On the other hand, as threads of the Silhouette Soft® have various vectors (Fig. 24.25), the position of the physician changes in various ways. Therefore, if the physician is not both handed, it is advisable to become familiar with the most comfortable position for the procedure.

Tip for the Silhouette Soft® Technique: Recommended Position for the Procedure

- Angle technique
  - Rt. horizontal suture → From the top of the patient's head
  - Lt. horizontal suture → From the left of patient's face
  - Rt/Lt vertical suture → From the right of patient's face
- PMA technique (U technique)
  - Rt → From the right side of the patient's face
  - Lt → From the left side of the patient's face
- Necklace technique (treatment for double chins)
  - Rt → From the side of the right shoulder of the patient
  - Lt → From the top of the patient's head

Prevention and Treatment of the Entry Point Dimple (Fig. 24.26)

- Causes
  - When an entry point hole is not sufficiently procured.
  - In inserting a needle, it does not go into the original hole perpendicularly but inserted in other direction.
- Prevention
  - Make the hole bigger than the needle diameter in making an entry point: Using an 18G needle or awl, perform dissection/revolving/subcision.

- A needle goes in perpendicularly.

  Until the black line enters to the skin level which is marked at the end of the needle (5 mm location), it should keep the originally procured hole (viz., it shall enter smoothly without resistance up to the black line). In such case, do not pinch too strongly, and pinch softly so that the originally procured hole exposes well.
- Treatment
  - Dissect the space the dermis/subcutaneous with the disinfected curved scissors.

In case you need to solve through molding (massage) in f/u after performing a Silhouette Soft® procedure

- Clear abnormality (e.g., severe unevenness in the left and right).
- Pain or asymmetry when the mouth opens widely.
- When the skin is pushed upward and downward using the hand, something hard is palpable or a dimple appears.

**Tip!**
When the Patient Complains that the Cone Is Touched at the Procedure Site

This is claimed mainly within several days after the procedure; sensing cones along the route of the thread when touched at the initial stage is not problematic.

**Fig. 24.26** Cause and prevention of dimple after the Silhouette Soft® procedure. When a thread is inserted in a straight line, a dimple does not occur at the entry point, but in techniques where the direction of the thread changes, cautions must be taken against dimples at the entry point. In the technique like (**b**), dimples can occur a lot at the red dot area (entry point). The first figure in (**a**) shows insertion of needle into an entry point. If the route is procured along the direction of the thread when making an entry point like in the second figure, dimples can be prevented (see Fig. 43.9). (©Medbook Co., Ltd. All rights reserved)

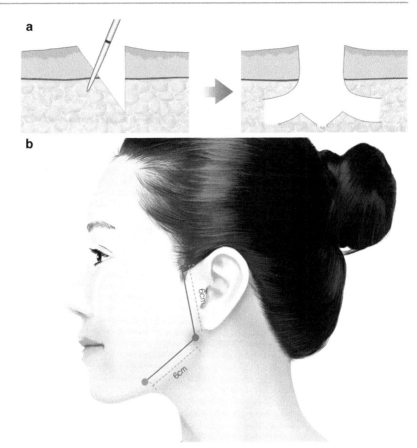

**Summary**
Various Tips for the Silhouette Soft® Procedures

- Method of holding a needle
  - In holding a needle, use the middle of the distal phalanx with the thumb and the index finger.
  - Depending on the case, sometimes the needle must be held by the tip of the fingers closely to the nails.
- In passing a needle
  - Depth
  - Direction of the bevel
  - The other hand: pinch or press
- For preventing dimples at the entry point
  - Dissection (disinfected scissors).
  - Dissect the space between the dermis and the subcutaneous layer with spring scissors.

- Position of the procedure for U technique
  - Rt → From the right side of the patient's face
  - Lt → From the left side of the patient's face
- Necklace technique (treatment for double chins)
  - Rt → From the side of the patient's right shoulder
  - Lt → From above the patient's head

Side effects after Silhouette Soft® procedure

- Suture rupture
- Temporary entry point dimple
- Skin fold
- Bruise
- Hematoma

## 25.1 Temporal Muscle Hypertrophy (or Trigonocephaly)

If the temporal muscle is well developed or the shape of the skull has a wide horizontal width due to the trigonocephaly (so-called bulging head-temporal area), a long cannula insertion may face interference in its progression.

Namely, after a cannula enters into an entry point, it must proceed at a consistent depth of the subcutaneous layer, but in such case, as the cannula tilts, it may go more deeply than intended gradually, resulting in inadvertent penetration of the fascia up to the muscle layer.

- **Solution**
- Rather than gripping the end of the cannula, it is helpful to grip as closely as possible to the entry point in proceeding at a consistent depth within the tissues.

## 25.2 Temporal Hollowness

If a temple area is sunken, a situation which is directly opposite from the temporal muscle hypertrophy occurs. In this area, a cannula passes more superficially than usual (intended). On the contrary, before zygomatic arch area, it tends to pass through the deeper area so that it can touch a mus-

cle. Especially, if it is accompanied by zygomatic arch prominence, this can be even more severe.

- **Solution**
  - If a tumescent solution or diluted lidocaine is injected using a cannula sufficiently in to the subcutaneous layer, the hollowness is adjusted, and passage of the cannula will be easy.
  - If the temporal hollowness is corrected first using fillers, passaging a cannula becomes easy.

## 25.3 Zygomatic Bone Prominence

Zygomatic bone is rather developed in Asian faces. When you want to proceed a cannula or a needle from the temple area toward the anterior cheek through zygomatic bone prominence, it is not easy to pass at a constant depth because it must pass a severe curve. Also, as this area has little fat and is dense, more force is needed in passing through with a cannula.

- **Solution**
  - By passing while holding a cannula or needle to bend, going along the curve becomes easy.
  - It is also a good method to avoid curves when designing insertion routes.

© Springer Nature Singapore Pte Ltd. 2019
B. Kim et al., *The Art and Science of Thread Lifting*, https://doi.org/10.1007/978-981-13-0614-3_25

## 25.4  Sunken Cheek

Sunken cheek stands out more as people grow older mostly. It is considered to make a charming face in Western country, but Asian women tend not to like this. To correct this area, fillers are sometimes used. In case of effective thread lifting, they can achieve not only lower face lifting but also correction of this sunken part.

This area requires thorough understanding of anatomical structure. It consists of the zygomatico-cutaneous ligament and the masseteric cutaneous ligament; it forms a diamond or triangular shape (see Fig. 44.2). Sagging faces have vectors toward the inferior or the medial side in general, but this part faces toward the inner (deeper) side (inner vector; see Fig. 22.13). This area is one of the densest tissues in the face. Therefore, in this area, insertion depth cannot be controlled while passing a cannula, and much force is exerted to pass. Also this area is not lifted well even by pinching using fingers. When a thread penetrates the very center of this area, dimples or distortion of the skin (abnormal hanging by cogs) occurs well (see Fig. 44.3).

- **Solution**
  - In designing, it must be designed in a way not to pass through the very center of the sunken cheek. (Depending on the type of the thread, a skillful practitioner may avoid this side effects even though the thread

passes through the very center. But it is advisable for beginners to avoid this area in designing.)
- If the thread passes the side of the sunken cheek area (diamond shape), passing becomes easy, and the likelihood of side effects can be reduced.
- However, if the procedure is performed totally away from this area, the remaining area would be lifted well, and this area would not be lifted well, which may appear somewhat lacking. In such case, by inserting one to two short-/medium-sized cog thread(s) to be hung up to the middle of the sunken cheek in the last stage of the procedure, it can have beneficial effects, and occurrence of dimples can be reduced.
- As this area is not pinched well, it is advisable to press with fingers instead. If this area is pressed by using the two or three fingers of the opposite hand while the cannula or needle passes, it passes more easily.
- **Cautions**
  - It is advisable to have the patient acknowledge existing sunken cheek prior to the procedure. This is because in some cases, the patient claims that sunken cheek which did not exist appeared after procedure as the patient did not recognize it before.

## 25.5  Operation Scar: Zygomatic Bone Reduction Surgery, Double-Jaw Surgery, and Lifting Surgery

If there are remaining scars due to surgery on the insertion route of thread, it is not easy for a cannula or needle to pass. Sometimes, even a needle cannot pass well, and the skin is pushed toward the direction of the progression during thread insertion. Prior to the procedure, it is necessary to check a history of operation and to observe carefully whether there is any scar during designing process. Sometimes, patients hide prior surgical experiences. In addition to the suture scars which are visible, it is also necessary to inspect whether there is a tissue adhesion on the insertion route within subcutaneous tissues, which can make a cannula difficult to pass.

- **Solution**
  - In designing, the scar areas must be avoided.
  - When a cannula or a needle does not pass well, it can pass more easily by pressing these areas with fingers

## 25.6   Liposuction

Patients who have undergone a liposuction on the face have more fibrotic facial fat tissue than average person. In such case, as it affects passing of cannula, inserting a cannula is not easy.

- **Solution**
  - When a cannula or a needle does not pass well, pressing the tissues using the second and third fingers of opposite hand is useful to pass.
  - When holding a cannula, it is easier to control the force by gripping the tip of cannula.

## 25.7   Acne Scars

If patients have severe rolling scars or boxcars among types of acne scars, the bottom of the scars have fibrotic connections with the subcutaneous tissues. When passing this area, they can make a cannula or a needle hard to pass.

- **Solution**
  - When a cannula or needle does not pass well, pressing the tissues using the second and third fingers of opposite hand is useful to pass.

## 25.8   History of Lifting Procedure: Thread Lifting and HIFU

In many cases patients considered the interval of thread lifting treatment as 1 year. In such case, the patients undergo a fibrotic change in subcuta-

neous fat tissues by previous thread insertion. It is likely to meet resistance when a cannula or needle passes the tissues.

Also, there are many patients who got HIFU treatment several months before. In such case, facial fat tissues generally get a fibrotic change. Likewise, this affects passing of a cannula or a needle.

- **Solution**
  - When a cannula or a needle does not pass well, pressing the tissues using the second and third fingers of the opposite hand is useful to pass.

**Summary**

Difference in Density of Fat Tissues Depending on the Facial Area (Fig. 25.1)

- Fat is non-fibrotic from the temple to the zygomatic arch.
- When passing the zygomatic arch, it is fibrotic.
- The sunken cheek is the most fibrotic.
- After passing the sunken cheek, fat becomes soft.
- It becomes more fibrotic as it is closer to the medial cheek.

**Summary**

Prognostic Factors that Affect the Outcome of Thread Lifting: Checkpoints to Predict the Prognosis Prior to the Procedure

1. Masseter Muscle Hypertrophy
   If a patient has a square jaw due to a masseter muscle hypertrophy, even though simulation of lifting vector is done with hands prior to the procedure, lifting effect is minimal.
   - Solution
     - To correct a square jaw, pretreatment using the botulinum toxin is

**Fig. 25.1** Area where passing of a cannula/ needle is demanding (areas with dense connective tissues)

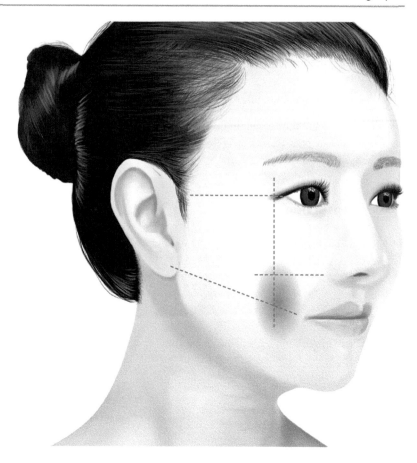

needed. toxin, it is most effective to perform the lifting procedure in 1 to 2 months, when the effect of the reduction of the square jaw is produced. However, in reality, the botulinum toxin treatment is done together on the same day as the thread lifting procedure in many cases.

– When explaining a patient the before and after effects of the procedure, rather showing the front, show the side, emphasizing the cleared jaw line and the corrected jowl and marionette line. During the explanation with a frontal view, lifting simulation does hardly make a square jaw to become a V-line.

2. Amount of the Whole Cheek Fat/ Sagging of Localized Fat
   • When treating patients with a lot of fat in the cheek, as more pulling force is required, the lifting effect may be reduced.
   • In that case, it can be solved by using long threads rather than short threads or increasing the number of short threads.
   • If there is sagging of the localized fat, such as the jowl and the marionette line, the lifting effect is kind of good.
3. Degree of Sagging of the Marionette Line/Jowl
   • In case that a patient has a mild to moderate sagging of the marionette line or the jowl, it is proper to make a lifting effect. Prior to the procedure,

it is useful to show the expected result by simulating in the mirror.

4. Amount of Submandibular Fat
   - If a patient has a double chin, favourable effects can be expected by using long bidirectional threads. In the past, liposuction was performed to correct a double chin, but it can be treated only through a simple thread lifting procedure. In performing a lower face lifting procedure, the chin contour becomes clearer if the procedure is performed with submandibular fat lifting.

**Summary**

A Checklist to Explain Patients Prior to the Procedure

1. Checking Elevation of Lateral Canthus
   - In inserting a thread from the mandible, passing the zygomatic arch and toward the temple, elevation of the lateral canthus can occur if the most medial thread is close to the lateral canthus (see Fig. 23.4). Most patients do not want the elevation of the lateral canthus after a lifting procedure. This is because it can make them look fierce. There are some young patients who want the lateral canthus to be elevated. In which case, the desired result can be obtained by designing the most medial thread to be more medial than the normal design. As most patients do not want this, it is necessary to check this prior to the procedure showing the mirror and to keep 2FB (fingerbreadth) in distance between the most medial thread and the lateral canthus.

2. Showing a Simulation of Expected Result
   - As explained in Part 5–1, in performing a thread lifting, the most favorable vectors are the one from the marionette line to the earlobe/from the mandible, passing the zygomatic arch and toward the temple/from the nasolabial folds passing the zygomatic arch toward the hairline, etc. Prior to the procedure, decide the optimal vector with simulation using a mirror. In pulling the skin with the fingers, it is easy for patients to understand if the explanations about the difference in the types and numbers of threads are provided by differing the number of fingers. As the vector considered by the physician can be different from outcome desired by the patient, this process is necessary prior to the procedure (see Part 1 – Design and Patient's Choice).

3. Explaining Downtime of Entry Point/Hairline Shaving
   - Sites of entry points can be largely divided into three categories.
     ① Side of the face (hairline or behind the ears)
       - As the entry point is not easily seen, patients feel less discomfort, and it is convenient to disinfect before procedure.
     ② Location which can be exposed in front view (medial to the hairline)
       - Although disinfection is convenient, in case of large entry point hole, as it is easily exposed, it can cause discomfort.
     ③ Temple area (located on the scalp, inside hairline)
       - If the entry point is located on the scalp, there is the advantage of not being exposed perfectly. But disinfection and preparations prior to the procedure are complicated, and hair cutting is inevitable.
         – Usually cut about three to five hairs for each entry point (to minimize the number of hairs cut), which does not cause discomfort to the

      patient. In such case, if the hair around the entry point sticks out, it may interfere with the procedure. Therefore, it is mandatory to prepare the hair tightly with tools (see Fig. 23.7).

- In some cases, the hair around the entry point is shaved not to be tangled. As the interfering factors disappear, it is convenient for the practitioner, but it must be explained to the patient in advance and needs consent.

4. Checking Asymmetry
   - Most patients have asymmetry to a certain extent in their faces. But some patients are concerned about their asymmetry. In such cases, the sagged side is lifted more to correct asymmetry.
   - However, sometimes, patients and physicians do not realize the existing asymmetry of the face prior to the procedure, and patients claim that the procedure results in the asymmetry. Even if it is explained to the patient that the asymmetry existed before, the patients do not accept it well. Therefore, when designing, it is necessary to check thoroughly if there is any asymmetry.
   - Some patients want a perfect correction of severe asymmetry. In such case, it is advisable that the physician explain the patient honestly the expected result showing in the mirror. And it is necessary to pay attention to lift more the sagged side during the procedure.

# Part VII

# Procedures for Each Area

# Forehead (Eyebrows)

**Considerations**

The forehead area has small amount of soft tissues, and wrinkles are created by expressions in the frontalis muscle. To lift the top part of the forehead, the following considerations must be made.

- It is advisable to numb the function of the muscles which lower the forehead downward. Simultaneous use of botulinum toxin helps.
- Supplementing the volume and adjusting the hollowness in the wrinkle area must be considered.
- It is difficult to pull the forehead through simple lifting. Prior to the thread lifting, by dissecting soft tissues, it is necessary to pull the entire forehead upward.
- Forming a fixing point is more difficult in the forehead area than other areas.

If the effect is not satisfactory after the initial procedure, additional procedures must be considered. Also, toxin treatments on the frontalis muscle must be considered in addition.

1. Type of Thread
   - QT lift/Blue Rose Forte/ VOV(short cannula and inner needle)
   - Silhouette Soft®/silk heart
2. Thread Insertion
   - Insertion (driving) depth
   - Subcutaneous (above muscles)
   - Below muscles
   - Depth of anchoring: under the muscle
3. Considerations for Side Effects
   - Bleeding
     - Bleeding in the forehead lifting procedure occurs more often than in the cheek lifting procedure. In designing entry points, exits, and progression of threads, it is advisable not to overlap with blood vessels.
     - For preventing bleeding
       - Use a cannula over a needle.
       - Using a cannula in the driving route of the thread, anesthetize with lidocaine including epinephrine.
       - In designing, set a location by observing and avoiding the blood vessels.
   - Headache
     - In general, pain is experienced after the procedure up to around one week
     - Perform a combined botulinum toxin treatment routinely to the frontalis/corrugator muscle and prescribe the NSAID together.
4. Combined Treatment
   - Botulinum toxin
   - Filler
   - HIFU

© Springer Nature Singapore Pte Ltd. 2019
B. Kim et al., *The Art and Science of Thread Lifting*, https://doi.org/10.1007/978-981-13-0614-3_26

**Summary**

Simulation Prior to the Procedure (Frontalis Pulling/Traction Test)

- Perform simulation by showing a mirror to the patient prior to the procedure, and the degree of the effect must be understood. When the frontalis muscle is pulled upward pressing near the hairline, people whose eyebrows lift have the anatomical structure in which the frontalis muscle reacts in constant direction from the hairline to below the eyebrow.
- On the other hand, when the frontalis muscle is pulled upward pressing near the hairline, people whose eyebrows do not lift much have the anatomical structure in which the reactions above and below the frontalis muscle based on the center of the forehead are separate (probably, it is thought to have developed in the fascia at the middle point of the frontalis muscle or attached to the bone). In such case, when the skin is pulled upward from the center of the forehead, the eyebrows slightly lift. Therefore, for the patients who did not get satisfactory results from the frontalis pulling/traction test prior to the procedure, prior explanations are advisable.
- Lifting eyebrow lines and lifting drooped double eyelid lines should be considered separately. Until the mid-40s, when the eyebrows are lifted, the double eyelid lines elevate together, but if there is a skin laxity for those in the 50s or older, even the eyebrows are lifted, and changes to the double eyelid lines may be minimal, which needs to be confirmed to the patient as well.

**Fig. 26.1** Eyebrow lifting – simple fixing method. (Entry points and the number of threads to be inserted differ depending on the patients)

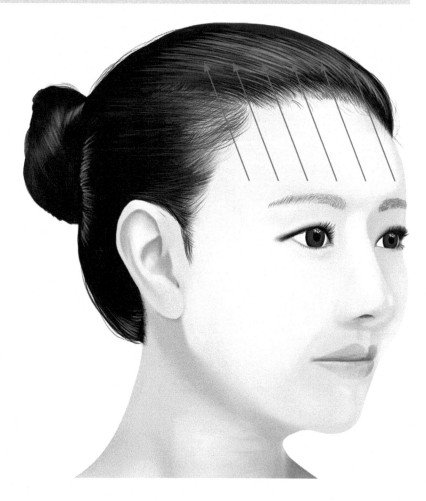

## 26.1    Simple Fixing Method (Fig. 26.1)

- Method of fixing by pulling the forehead with cogs.
- If there is a thick soft tissue including subcutaneous fat, the effect is also weak.
- If there are too little subcutaneous tissues, since they are conglutinated, pulling cannot be achieved.
- Lifting the forehead using the simple fixing method is insufficient.
- To display effects, supplemental procedures are required.
- After dissecting the loose connective tissue layer below the muscles of the forehead, pull upward using cog threads. Additional insertion of spike form threads would be helpful to prevent sagging down.
- A number of threads is necessary and dissection in an accurate layer is required.
- When using the above dissecting method, some effects may be expected also for the patients who have forehead tissues with strong conglutination.

## 26.2    X-Cross Method (Fig. 26.2)

- The X-cross method is a more effective lifting method fixing the forehead skin and the subcutaneous tissues.

**Fig. 26.2** Eyebrow lifting – X-cross method. (Designing must differ depending on the patients)

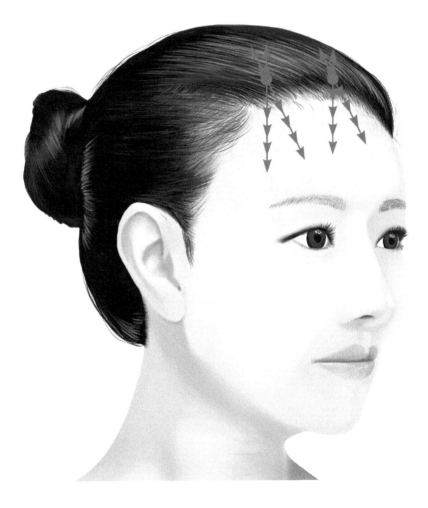

- After fixing through knotting, with the function of the cog in the opposite direction, it has the function of preventing the pulled skin from sagging down.
- There is lifting effect only if the pulled skin can drive above the insertion hole level.
- Instead of cutting and removing the opposite cogs, additional fixation can be achieved by inserting the remaining threads into the scalp.

## 26.3  Anchoring Method (Fig. 26.3)

1. Anatomy
   - Be careful with the STA (supratrochlear artery) or SOA (supraorbital artery): it passes the eyebrows and comes out of the subcutaneous layer.

- Check driving in the lateral – SV(sentinel vein), SfTA(superficial temporal artery), and SfTV (superficial temporal vein) (if checked while lying down, blood vessels show better).
- Dispersion of the frontalis muscle.

2. Designing
   - Near the curvature of the frontal bone: in inserting a cannula, set an entry point and exit where the curves are minimized.
   - If the patient's hairstyle normally exposes the forehead, set the entry point above the hairline so as not to expose the entry point.
   - The end of the thread at the exit point is on the corrugator muscle or the muscle fiber.
   - The number of threads differs depending on the degree of sagging.

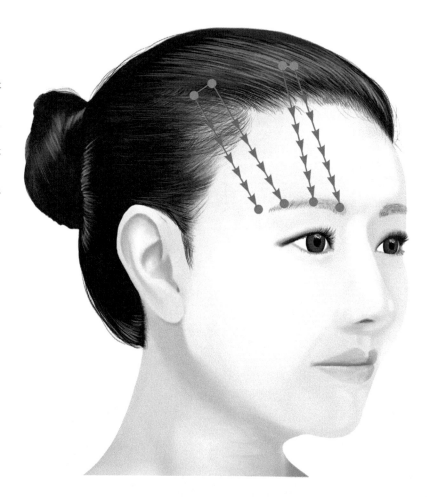

**Fig. 26.3**  Eyebrow lifting – Anchoring method. (In many cases, anchoring must be done inside the hairline, and it must be done in the area where the thread can drive in a straight line as much as possible. If there is a severe curve, it is difficult for the thread to progress, and the likelihood of side effects is high)

When lifting the forehead using the anchoring method, aging changes must be well understood. In general, as the skin around the eyes and the eyebrows are laxed, lifting of the lateral part is important.

It is recommended to insert and pass the thread in a deeper layer while performing forehead lifting. Caution must be taken to avoid unevenness and bumpiness due to a thin tissue coverage in the forehead. When lifting procedure is done on the lateral side of the face, it is important to bear in mind and avoid injury to major arteries and nerves

As nerve pathway is also mostly in the superficial layer in the area where the threads are inserted, deep-layer lifting is safe, provided, in the case of the procedure of the lateral part, sagging of the eyebrows may occur by damage to the facial nerve zygomatic branch.

## 27.1 Summary of the Eye Area Lifting

### 27.1.1 Lifting of the Eye Area

Laxity of the skin and the soft tissues in the eye areas is severe. The factor which must be decided foremost in treating the eye area is to check whether the patient is the adequate subject of the procedure. Lifting which uses absorbable threads are not fundamentally surgical; therefore, the process of removing the skin or soft tissues is not involved. Accordingly, a surgical effect cannot be expected.

Through simulation, the degree which can be improved through the absorbable thread lifting must be clearly explained. Satisfaction will decrease when the procedure is performed on a patient whose effect is hardly expected. The patient may need to get additional surgical treatments. In pulling with threads, many cases require dissection of tissues.

Reasons for considering surgical treatments first for lifting of the eye area compared to other areas are as follows:

- In general, the mechanism of lifting is evenly pulling the tissues below a certain fixing point in the head.
- Compared to this, the eye area tends to have more laxity in the skin and the soft tissues of the eyelids and the eye area than the forehead outside. Namely, the areas which needs the most pulling are the eye area and the eyelids rather than the forehead. Therefore, if it is pulled by a certain length around the eye area, this does not result in a sufficiently satisfactory result compared to the forehead area.
- To the contrary, as surgical methods directly removes the excessive tissues of eye area and the eyelids which have the most severe laxity, a better result can be obtained.

## 27.2 Anatomy of the Eye Area

### 27.2.1 Anatomy

In performing an absorbable thread lifting procedure to elevate the eye area, it is advisable to insert the thread into the supra-periosteal plane in the frontalis m. area and into the subcutaneous fat layer in the temporalis m. area.

Due to the possibility of damage in the superficial temporal vessels, bleeding must be minimized by using the pinch technique (Fig. 27.1).

The frontal branch of the facial n. forms many smaller branches (Fig. 27.2), and therefore, unless they are damaged all at once, nerve damage to the extent of raising clinical problems does not occur easily. However, the insertion layer must always be clearly understood and controlled smoothly to avoid nerve and vessel damage.

© Springer Nature Singapore Pte Ltd. 2019
B. Kim et al., *The Art and Science of Thread Lifting*, https://doi.org/10.1007/978-981-13-0614-3_27

**Fig. 27.1** Pathway of the STA. (Published with kind permission of © Kwan-Hyun Youn 2018. All rights reserved)

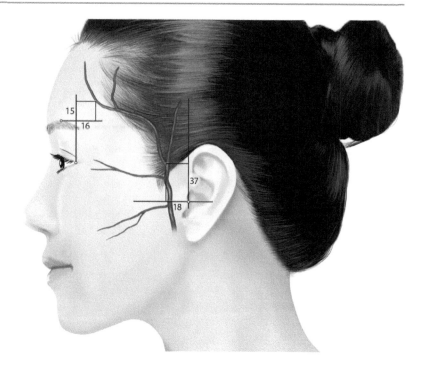

**Fig. 27.2** Facial nerve temporal branch. (Published with kind permission of © Kwan-Hyun Youn 2018. All rights reserved)

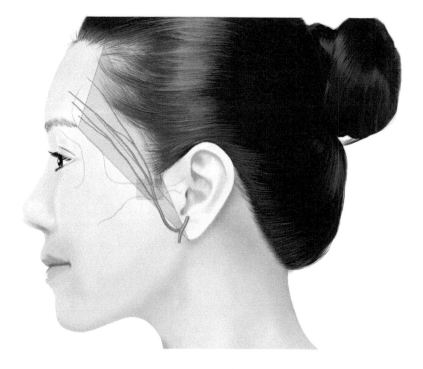

## 27.3 Techniques Which Can Be Used in the Eye Area

### 27.3.1 Preconditioning by Dissection with Tumescent Technique

As a method which can be applied to certain areas only, there is a technique by tumescent dissection.

Lifting using threads can be approached from two perspectives. Firstly, it is a method of directly pulling tissues using a thread. This is a method used in all areas and is a fundamental model.

Secondly, this is a method of fixing by using the thread after dissecting a specific layer of the tissue and pulling the tissues along the surface of dissection. Even before inserting the thread, this tumescent dissecting method causes lifting to occur naturally from dissecting and pulling. Provided, if pulled tissues are not fixed, the lifting effect disappears immediately. Namely, this is a method of dissecting a specific layer using the tumescent and fixing the area by inserting a cog thread.

This makes inserting of absorbable threads convenient, and it has been experienced that this reduced pain and bleeding. An objective study on the effect and duration of this technique is expected to be searched. Because, when a PDO (which is an absorbable thread ingredient) meets the tumescent which includes saline solution, there is a possibility that decomposition accelerates; this would be a very important study. In case of the authors, when we actually perform the procedure, after performing layer dissection through the tumescent solution, a post processing is performed in which the tumescent solution is squeezed with hands and removed.

### 27.3.2 Method of Forming a Fixing Point in the Eye Area

**Forming a fixing point**
- Fix using bi-directional cogs
- Fix using the tying method
- Combination of tying method and X-cross method for fixation with bi-directional cogs
- Fascia anchoring method

The tying method and the X-cross method are used a lot around the eye area.

### 27.3.3 Tying Method or Simple Cog Insertion Method (Fig. 27.3)

- The effect on the eye area is better when it is pulled farther away.
- To prevent the fierce impression by elevation of lateral canthus area only, it is recommendable to pull after performing wide hydro-dissection using tumescent solution.
- The layer of hydro-dissection is the layer below the frontalis m. in the forehead area and the layer between the deep temporal fascia and the superficial temporal fascia or the subcutaneous fat layer in the temple areas.
- If the cog thread is inserted and pulled after dissection, tissues are much more easily pulled than when there is no dissection.
- For fixing afterward, it can be helpful to use a thread in a spike form additionally.
- If sufficient dissection is done, fixing by inserting many spike threads only without bi-directional cogs is also effective.

### 27.3.4 X-Cross Method (Fig. 27.4)

- Similarly with the tying method, this is a method of inserting the remaining thread into the scalp instead of cutting and removing the opposite cogs after tying.
- As a function of cogs in opposite direction, longer and stronger effect can be expected.
- Basically, also around the eye area, the soft tissues are not easily lifted; lifting through hydro-dissection is recommended.
- In case of the X-cross technique, it is important to fix the cogs on opposite directions.
- For lifting, pulled skin must have gathered somewhere.
- As it is good to have the skin gather above the entry point, for this, insertion of the cog in an opposite direction must be done so that the cogs in the top hold the skin well.

**Fig. 27.3** Lifting the
eye area – tying method.
(This is a method which
can be used on patients
whose eye area wrinkles
can be improved by
slightly elevating the
skin in the eye area and
the temple area)

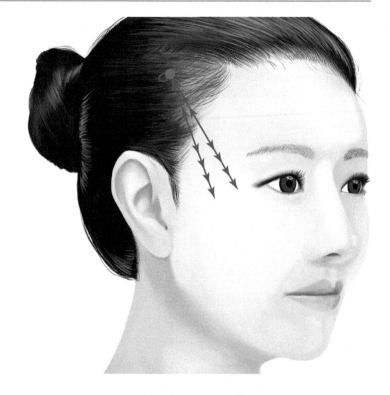

**Fig. 27.4** Lifting the
eye area – X-cross
method. The fixing point
can be formed more
strongly

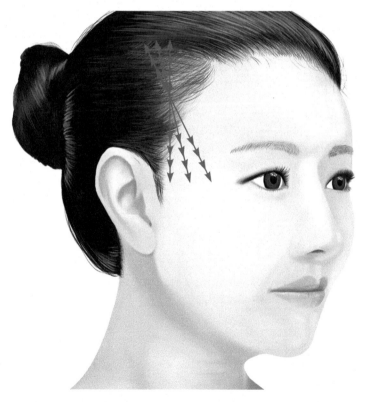

## 27.4 Cautions

The eye area lifting is a procedure that lifts both the lateral part of forehead and temple area simultaneously. Therefore, procedures are done in two areas which have anatomical difference. To be safe, the anatomical structure, blood vessel pathway and depth, and nerve pathway and depth must be all understood for both sides. At the same time, a combination treatment with botulinum toxin for muscle hyperactivity should also be taken.

However, the more important than anything else is not to cause wasting by unnecessarily recommending thread lifting procedures to patients who need surgical treatments.

## Considerations
Lower Cheek Lifting

- Making a suitable fixing point affects lifting outcomes in this area especially.
- The lower cheek is an area where sagging of fats and laxity of fibrotic tissues are severe as aging progresses.
- If the fixing point is weak, the effect is minimal or duration is short.
- It is important to select the method of forming fixing points depending on the condition of the patient.

Forming Fixing Points

- As V-line lifting using bi-directional cog threads has weak fixating ability, it has less effect and shorter efficacy in patients with more subcutaneous fat in the lower cheek.
- For patients who have thin tissue coverage in the face, satisfactory results can be obtained even just with a simple cog thread insertion or tying method.
- For those whose skin in the lower cheek is laxed or has excessive fat, forming strong fixing points is essential. The fascia anchoring method is necessary.
- Considering the folding phenomenon of the skin which necessarily occurs in forming fixing points, it is advisable to make entry points above the hairline as much as possible.

## 28.1 Fascia Anchoring Method (Fig. 28.1)

- This is the most strong and effective lifting.
- The technique is complicated and cautions must be taken in consideration of avoiding injury to blood vessels and nerves. Anatomical structure and technique must be well understood.
- It is a true lifting technique not just tightening.
- An entry point should be made inside the hairline not to show the pulled skin because pulled skin nearby anchoring area can be gathered around the entry point.
- Proceeding in a consistent layer is important to avoid dimpling of the skin.

**Fig. 28.1**  V-line lifting – fascia anchoring method using long threads This is the most important lifting procedure skill

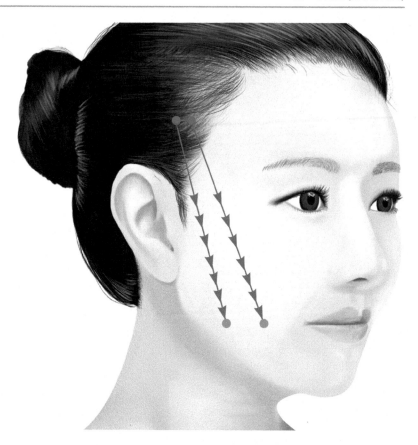

- Dimple can occur in the exit area where the thread comes out and can be resolved by taking adequate procedure.

## 28.2   Tying Method (Fig. 28.2)

- Pulling force is not so strong and the lifting method is similar to the function of gathering bi-directional cogs.
- The skin and the subcutaneous layer gather at the middle point of the bi-directional cogs.
- If the gathering point is not adjusted well, it causes the zygomatic arch to appear prominent, reducing satisfaction.
- It is not a powerful lifting method, so its effect would be restricted on people with lots of subcutaneous fat in the lower cheek and thick tissue coverage.
- Its effect is good on people who have thin skin and less subcutaneous fat.

- Selecting the right patient is important, and if suitable patients are chosen, it can be done easily, and the result is also good.
- It is necessary to insert sufficient amount of threads.

## 28.3   X-Cross Method (Fig. 28.3)

- Basically, this technique is similar to the tying method.
- By not cutting the cogs in the remaining area and pushing them toward the opposite direction, this strengthens the power of cogs in the fixing area.
- As the procedure is easy and it is stronger than the tying method, this is a preferred technique.
- As we can gather lifted skin to specific point, various designs are possible. It is useful to have it gather within the hair not to show it as much as possible, which requires skills accordingly.

**Fig. 28.2** V-line
lifting – tying method.
(It is relatively easy and
has favorable effects.
Designing is important.
It is advisable to make
entry points at invisible
areas as much as
possible)

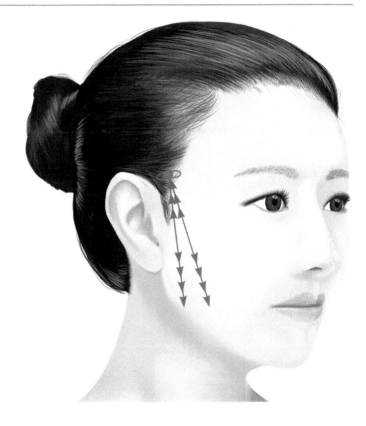

**Fig. 28.3**  V-line
lifting – X-cross method
Form stronger fixing
points

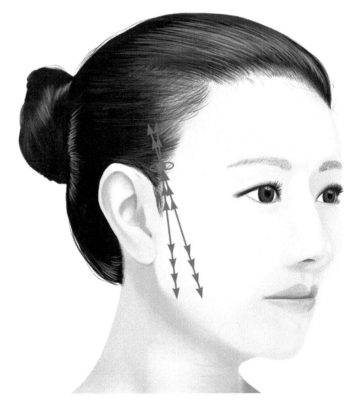

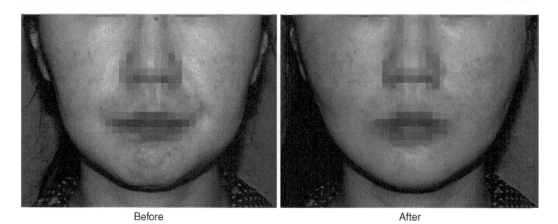

Before                                                          After

**Fig. 28.4** V-line lifting – before and after photos

**Considerations**

- Thread lifting and volumizing effects are considered simultaneously.
- Selecting fixing point is difficult.
- Pulling the fat layer above the nasolabial folds using bi-directional cogs. In such case, the zygomatic bone area can be enlarged due to the gathering function of the bi-directional cogs. Through diagnostic process, if zygomatic bone is expected to be widening after the procedure, other methods must be considered.

## 29.1 Anchoring Method (Fig. 29.1)

## 29.2 Method of Fixing with Bi-Directional Cogs
(Fig. 29.2)

© Springer Nature Singapore Pte Ltd. 2019
B. Kim et al., *The Art and Science of Thread Lifting*, https://doi.org/10.1007/978-981-13-0614-3_29

**Fig. 29.1** Nasolabial
fold lifting – anchoring
method. (Through
simulation, vectors must
be understood
accurately)

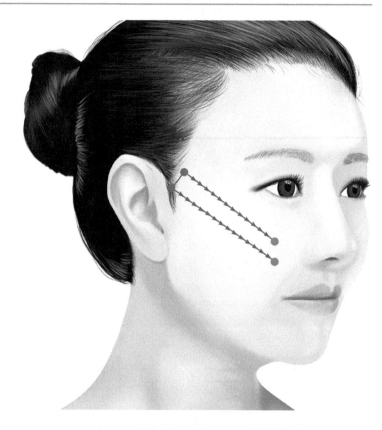

**Fig. 29.2** Nasolabial
fold lifting – techniques
with bi-directional cogs

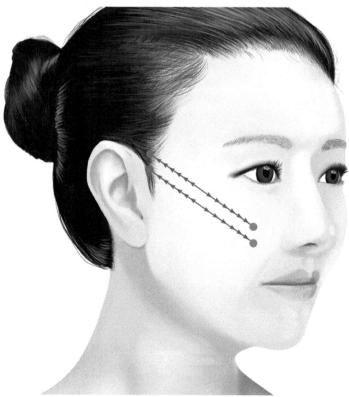

**Considerations**
- The marionette line must be designed considering the treatment of the lower cheek and jowl.
- Injecting fillers alone in the sunken area to soften the marionette line can aggravate the sagging of the face. The lower cheek area which makes the marionette line must be lifted toward the ear (Fig. 30.1).

- The procedure pulling the sagged lower cheek area upward must be considered with filler injection simultaneously.

- Wrinkles in the marionette area need to be pulled toward the ear.
- Due to the characteristics of lifting, if the skin is pulled, the pulled skin must be gathered somewhere.

**Fig. 30.1** Vectors of marionette line lifting. Simulation must be performed to test which pulling vector is effective. Then, understand the optimal vectors and design accordingly

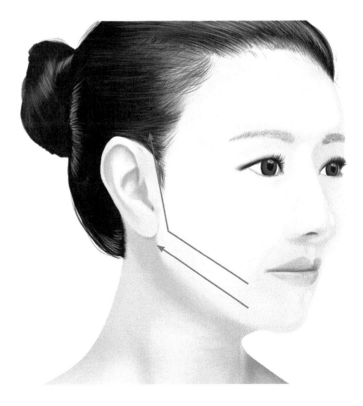

© Springer Nature Singapore Pte Ltd. 2019
B. Kim et al., *The Art and Science of Thread Lifting*, https://doi.org/10.1007/978-981-13-0614-3_30

- Some of the excessive skin gathers anterior to the ear, and the procedures must be done in detail to decrease the degree of the folds and wrinkles as much as possible.

- Skin dimpling inevitably occurs in the area of entry point marked in red dot; the degree of pulling must be controlled closely to minimize this.

## 30.1   Angle Technique (Fig. 30.2)

- After inserting the bi-directional cog thread in the entry point, bend the direction in the middle and progress to the marionette line area.
- The cogs in the marionette part play a pulling role, and the cogs in the head side play the role of fixing the pulled skin.
- An additional benefit of angle technique is to restore the sunken cheek area from the soft tissue gathering effect of bi-directional cogs.

## 30.2   L Shape Technique (Kim's Technique) (Fig. 30.3)

- The L shape technique is different to the angle technique; the two ends of the thread come out through the exit point in blue dot.
- Various types of cannula or long needle with threads can be used.
- Although it shows more effective tissue gathering and stronger lifting effects than the angle technique, this also requires detailed procedure as more wrinkles and dimple can result in the skin.

**Fig. 30.2** Marionette line lifting – angle technique. Lifting is performed by inserting the thread right above the zygomatic arch (red dot), bending in the lower area of the ear to proceed to the marionette area, removing the cannula, and pulling the thread

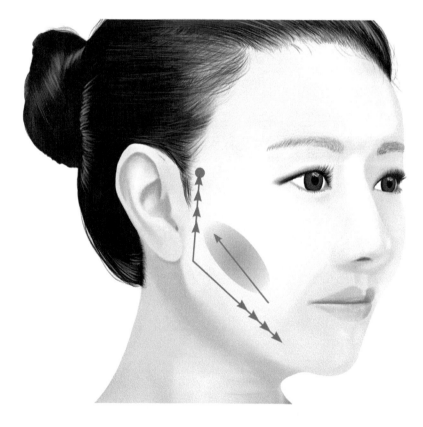

**Fig. 30.3** Marionette line lifting – L shape technique

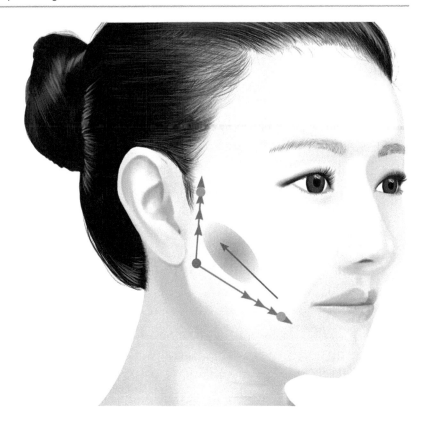

## 30.3 Anchoring Technique: Pulling Method Behind the Jaw Line (Fig. 30.4)

**Summary**
Setting an Entry Point Around the Mastoid Process

Bruising and Swelling
- This point is also used in performing double chin lifting.
- Pain may occur during or after the procedure.
- There are some people who have dense and thick surrounding tissues. In such case, it may be very difficult to make an entry point or to proceed with a cannula.
- If an experienced physician performs the procedure, a good outcome can be obtained but as beginners may experience difficulty with controlling pain, entry point dimples and driving of cannula. The procedure can be done easily without these problems if the entry point is set in the area where the skin is right behind the mandibular angle rather than mastoid process area (Post-Mandibular Anchoring Technique; see Fig. 24.19).

**Fig. 30.4** Marionette line lifting – anchoring technique – pulling method behind the jaw line. It is important to perform on suitable patients. If the patient group is selected after well understanding the contents in Part 5-1 Designing and Choice of Patients, good results can be expected. This is a very useful technique

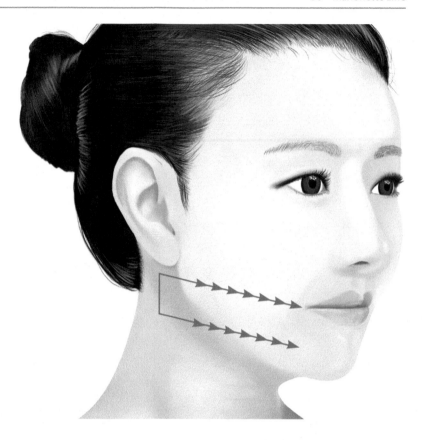

## 30.3.1 Designing

Entry point: set two entry points vertically in 1FB intervals (1.5 cm) behind the mandibular angle.

- If the sagging in the cheek area is severe, the effect of the angle technique or L shape technique may be insufficient.
- In such case, for more effective lifting, the pulling inevitably needs to be done from below the ear beyond the mandibular angle.
- It is recommended to perform lifting causing the skin to fold slightly using the anchoring method.

## 30.4   Tornado (Twister Thread) Supplementary Method (Fig. 30.5)

- If rigid and twisted spring form threads named "tornado" (twister) are inserted into the marionette area, the lower cheek and the marionette fold can be improved simultaneously.
- It may be the combined effect of denaturation of fat and tissue fibrosis
- The procedure is easy and simple. If the effect is insufficient after the procedure, other procedures must be considered in additional.

**Fig. 30.5** Marionette
line lifting – tornado
supplementary method.
This is a technique using
the characteristics of
thread of spring type.
Strictly speaking this is
not a lifting procedure

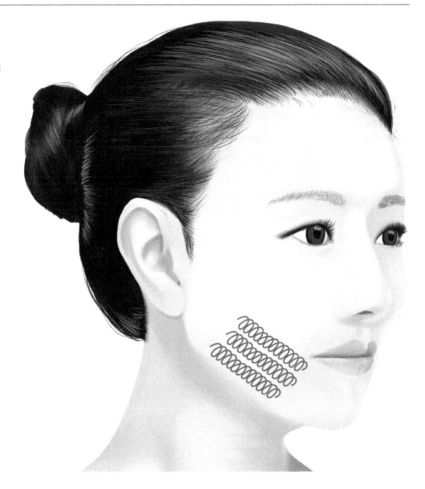

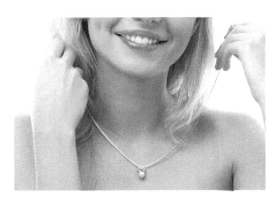

**Fig. 31.1** Lifting double chins – necklace technique

## Considerations

- This displays a good effect on patients whose excessive subcutaneous fat is the cause for the sagging of the neck.
- In case of those whose subcutaneous fat is thin, sinking and contracture occur highly.
- This is a technique which must be supported by the skill which can proceed evenly in the layer of the same depth along the facial and neck curves.
- Cautions must be taken against cases of bleeding and nerve damage. As the driving of the greater auricular nerve behind the ear is superficial, cautions must be taken.
- In passing the lower jaw area, cautions must be taken against damaging the salivary gland.
- Prior diagnosis is required to see whether the neck sagging is resulted from enlargement of the salivary gland.

- The difference in the locations of the skin and the subcutaneous fat layer when one is lying down and sitting down is large. Designing must be done when sitting down. The designing must be done in a way so that the thread does not pass up to the body of the mandible.

**Summary**
Mechanisms of the Necklace Technique

Mechanism of Lifting Double Chin Using the Necklace Technique
- By pulling the sagged fat in the center (Fig. a) toward both sides and lifting up muscles and deep fat, it is a mechanism of repositioning fat.
- Using 12 cones or 16 cones, set an entry point at the center and set an exit on both sides.
- This is a concept which is directly opposite to the technique which pulls from each of two sides using two threads. The direction of the cone is directly opposite compared to the technique which pulls from two sides.

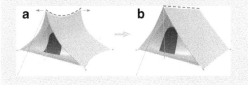

© Springer Nature Singapore Pte Ltd. 2019
B. Kim et al., *The Art and Science of Thread Lifting*, https://doi.org/10.1007/978-981-13-0614-3_31

## 31.1   Necklace Technique

### 31.1.1  Designing

- Entry point: set two entry points in 1FB (1.5 cm) interval in the center line of submental area.
- Exit: near the SCM (sternocleidomastoid muscle) – length of one side to be around 9 cm.

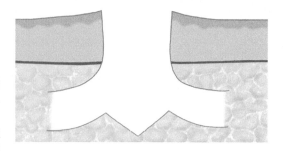

**Fig. 31.3**  Entry point

- If the exit is located more behind than the SCM, discomfort may be experienced from pulling during neck rotation movement.
- Moreover, tissue becomes denser as moving toward posterior area of the neck; therefore more force is required for passing a cannula or needle.

### 31.1.2  Making an Entry Point

• Make a sufficiently large hole using a puncture needle (because dimple frequently occurs).

### 31.1.3  Insertion

- Position: neck flexion makes double chins to be exposed.
- Depth: insert thread slightly deeper than the cheek area using the V-pinch technique (into deep subcutaneous tissue).

### 31.1.4  Traction and Cutting

- After thread insertion is completed, pull each half of the thread at both sides.
- (Pulling a right half of the thread by a right-handed person) While holding the end of the thread with the left hand, push the skin to the center of the chin with a snap using the thumb of the right hand. In such case, the assistance holds a left half of the thread so that it is not move.

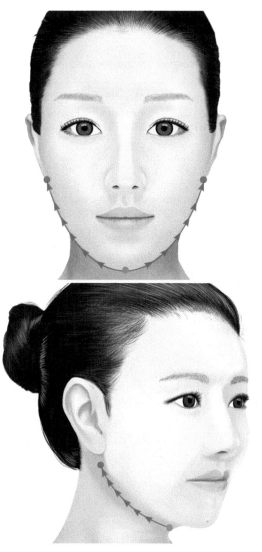

**Fig. 31.2**  Double chin lifting – design of necklace technique: entry point and exit point

**Fig. 31.4** Double chin lifting – design of necklace technique: entry point and exit point

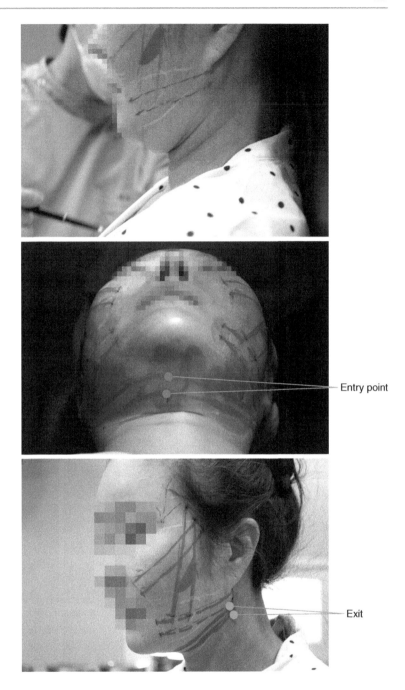

Entry point

Exit

## 31.1.5 Side Effects: Pain and Dimples

- Right after the procedure or the next day, patients claim stiffness in the submental area (feeling of pressing/embracing the neck).

- After 2–3/3–4 days, pain disappears (day 1, painful; day 3, slightly improves but still remains; day 4, pain disappears).
- If the patients feel stiff in the entry point, dimples are usually seen in this area.

**Fig. 31.5** Comparison of methods for double chin lifting. (**a**) Conventional technique: entry point located below both ears/exit located at the center. (**b**) Necklace technique: entry point located at the center/exit located on both sides

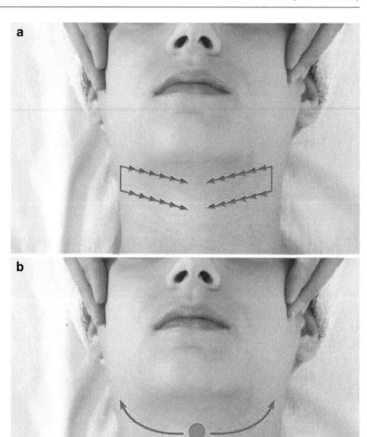

- If patients flex the neck after the procedure, entry point dimples can be easily seen. In case of severe dimples, it is necessary to dissect tissues between the subcutaneous fat and dermis and to explain to the patient. If left untreated, severe dimples are not spontaneously resolved with time.

### 31.1.6  Cautions in Choosing Patients

1. Indication (cases with good effect)
   - When a patient has a mild skin laxity and a moderate amount of fat
   - When double chins appear
   - When skin and fat thickness is 1.5 cm or more while pinching

2. Contraindication (cases with poor effect)
   - When there is severe skin laxity and little amount of fat (especially in old patients).
   - If skin laxity is severe like the Turkish neck, as the skin gathers in the center part of the neck, it can be more wrinkly.

### 31.1.7  Factors Which Affect the Outcome of the Procedure

1. When effects are good
   - If the curve connecting the entry point and the exit in both sides makes a smooth arc (Fig. 31.9a)

- If the depth of thread insertion is consistent and deep within the subcutaneous layer
2. When effects are poor
   - If the curve connecting the entry point and the exit in both sides makes a W shape (or seagull shape) (Fig. 31.9b)
     - In such case dimple frequently occurs at the entry point.
     - Using the conventional technique (Fig. 31.5a) may be a better choice rather than necklace technique.
   - If depth of the thread insertion is inconstant
     - The curve connecting the entry point and the two sides of the exit may be determined not only by designing of physicians but also by the condition of the patients (patients' factors – length of a mandibular body and angle between a horizontal line and a mandible body).

**Tip!**
Rather than inserting into the posterior to SCM (sternocleidomastoid muscle) by elongating the thread, it is important to proceed at a deep and constant depth of the subcutaneous layer!

It is necessary to explain possibility of dimple prior to the procedure to patients.

1. If the distance from the very center of the bi-directional thread to the cog/cone is too long, the effect of lifting at the very center of the chin may decrease. If insertion is done after making an additional knots at the center of the bi-directional threads, the lifting effect of the very center of the chin is better and duration becomes longer (in case of Silhouette Soft®).
2. Rather than setting the entry points of the two threads at the very center, if the entry point of the first thread is set slightly more to the left from the center line and the entry point of the second thread is set slightly more to the right from the center line, having only the thread at the very center of the double chins without any cog/cone can be avoided (in case of Silhouette Soft®).

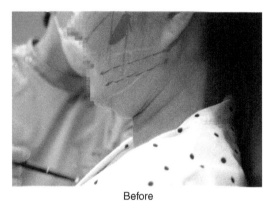
Before

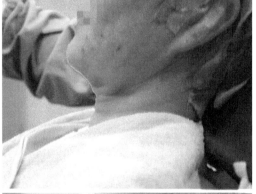

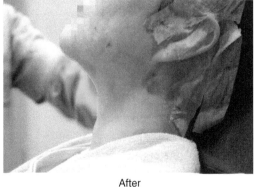
After

**Fig. 31.6** Double chin lifting – before and after (extension and flexion) photos of the necklace technique

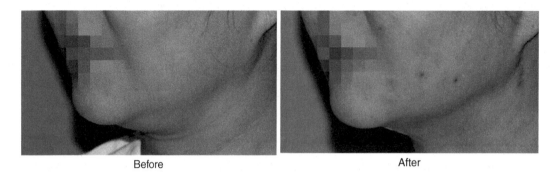

Before                                      After

**Fig. 31.7** Double chin lifting – before and after photos of the necklace technique. Two threads of the Silhouette Soft® (12 cones) were used for double chin lifting. There are two entry points at the center, and two exists below the ears

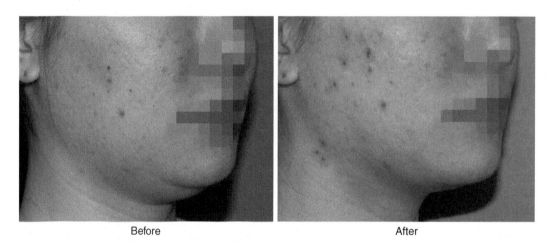

Before                                      After

**Fig. 31.8** Double chin lifting – before and after photos of the necklace technique

**Fig. 31.9** Relationship between dimple and design in performing the necklace technique. (**a**) Design which does not result in dimple. (**b**) Design which results in frequent occurrence of dimple (if this design is used, dimple occurs frequently as force gathers at the entry point which is at the very center of the thread as the figure in the right)

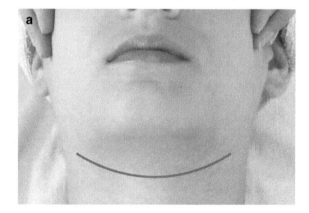

**Fig. 31.9** (continued)

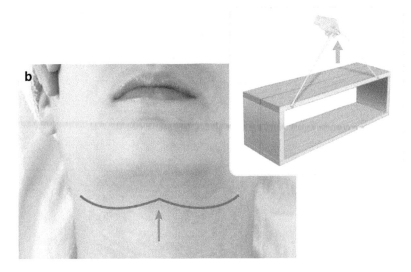

## 31.2 Method of Anchoring Below the Ear (Conventional Technique)

- This is a method of lifting by fixing near the mastoid behind the neck or dense subcutaneous tissues in the below.
- The lifting effect is strong, but sometimes it can cause severe pain.
- In some cases, the skin may fold a lot, but this is a hardly visible area.

## 31.3 Method of Combining the Neck: Marionette

- This technique can be used when it is necessary to treat the neck and the marionette line simultaneously.
- This is a method of lifting the neck and the lower cheek simultaneously using an anchoring method below the mastoid.
- Long threads must be used for anchoring method. In this case, tying technique using two bi-directional cogs is rarely used.

- Long Silhouette Soft® threads or long PDO threads (QT lift) are used. Lower mastoid area is an adequate fixing point as it is a lesion where tissue movement is limited.

## 31.4 Method of Tying or Simple Burying

- This is a method of lifting the skin and the subcutaneous fat in the laxed neck area using bi-directional cogs or unidirectional cogs.
- Effects are good when the skin is not thick and the amount of the subcutaneous fat is not much.
- In case there is lots of subcutaneous fat, the effects disappear quickly if the function of the fixing point is not strong.
- However, if the PDO dissolves and disappears, it causes fibrosis and contraction of surrounding tissues and stimulates the dermis; in some cases the best outcome shows after a period of times.
- Designing must be done while sitting up straight to prevent the thread from passing above the mandibular angle.

**Fig. 31.10** Double chin lifting – anchoring method

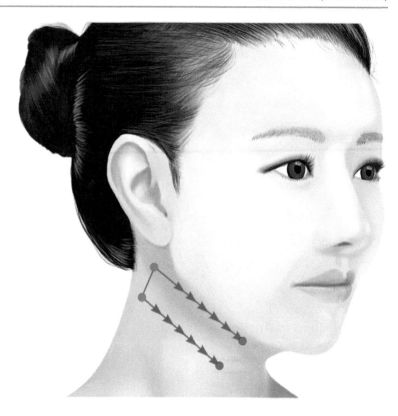

**Fig. 31.11** Double chin lifting – anchoring method (method of combining the neck and marionette)

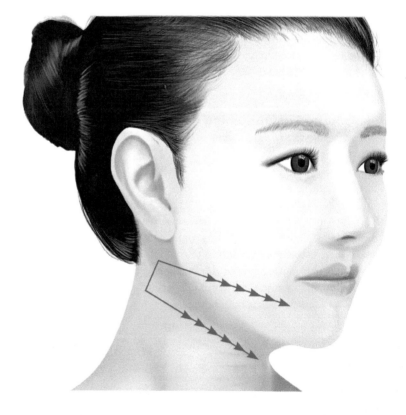

**Fig. 31.12** Double chin lifting – simple burying method

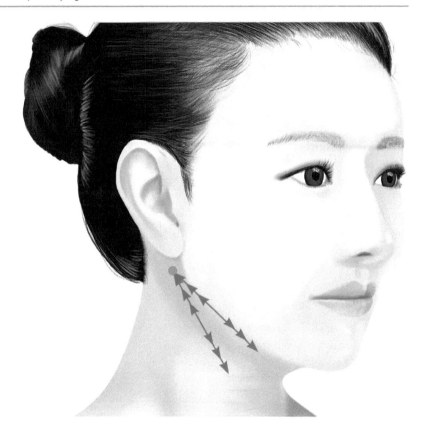

## 32.1 Method of Filling Wrinkles

- In many cases, horizontal wrinkles in the neck are difficult to solve.
- Even if the skin is pulled surgically, that is also difficult to solve.
- The cause of the occurrence of the horizontal wrinkles in the neck is reduction in the volume of the dermis and the subcutaneous layer. Therefore, if adequate volume is supplemented, neck wrinkles can be improved.
- However, the neck is thin skin and a lot of movement, it is not easy to make it completely disappear.
- By inserting threads which can fill in volume along the wrinkles, the wrinkles can be improved (Fig. 32.1).
- Strictly speaking this is filling rather than lifting.
- Rather than inserting the thread in the form of simple monofilament, by inserting mesh form threads, effects can be expected from the connective tissues growing and filling inside.
- To optimize the proliferation effects of the tissues, combining with various supplemental treatments can be considered.

© Springer Nature Singapore Pte Ltd. 2019
B. Kim et al., *The Art and Science of Thread Lifting*, https://doi.org/10.1007/978-981-13-0614-3_32

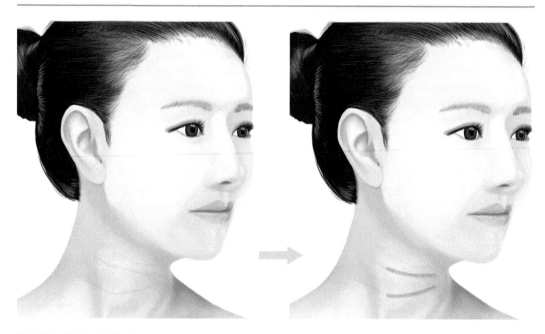

**Fig. 32.1** Neck wrinkle lifting method of filling wrinkles. Strictly speaking, this is not a lifting. This is a petit wrinkle cosmetic procedure using threads

# Part VIII

# Evaluation of Procedure Outcome

# Method of Evaluating the Effect of Thread Lifting

GAIS score is generally used for evaluation of thread lifting effect (Table. 33.1). The contents of the GAIS score are as follows:

When interpreting the GAIS score, you have to keep in mind two facts. Firstly, the smaller the number, the better effect it means. Secondly, the GAIS score does not evaluate the effect objectively, but tells the degree of improvement subjectively.

It would be nice to measure the effect of thread lifting through an evaluation tool that is objectively quantified. Although not perfect, the judgment method using the Morpheus which will be talked about later can be a solution to objective result evaluation.

**Table 33.1** Global Aesthetic Improvement Scale (GAIS)

| Degree | | Description |
|---|---|---|
| 1 | Exceptional improvement | Excellent corrective result |
| 2 | Very improved patient | Marked improvement of the appearance, but not completely optimal |
| 3 | Improved patient | Improvement of the appearance, better compared with the initial condition, but a touch-up is advised |
| 4 | Unaltered patient | The appearance substantially remains the same compared with the original condition |
| 5 | Worsened patient | The appearance has worsened compared with the original condition |

© Springer Nature Singapore Pte Ltd. 2019
B. Kim et al., *The Art and Science of Thread Lifting*, https://doi.org/10.1007/978-981-13-0614-3_33

## 34.1 Simulation Using Morpheus®

### 34.1.1 Evaluation of Outcomes

It is not easy to simulate soft tissue changes before and after the procedure by computer. However, due to technology development, this has become possible to a certain extent. In case of the Morpheus® equipment, we can simulate the changes in volume and soft tissue movement.

Figures 34.1 and 34.2 below show the simulation of midface thread lifting, frontal cheek filler, and chin filler using the Morpheus® equipment, comparing it to the result of the actual procedure.

### 34.1.2 Judging Outcomes

Figure 34.3 This figure shows the volume change after thread lifting, frontal cheek filler, and chin filler mentioned above using Morpheus®. These are virtual images of posttreatment by simulation using Morpheus system.

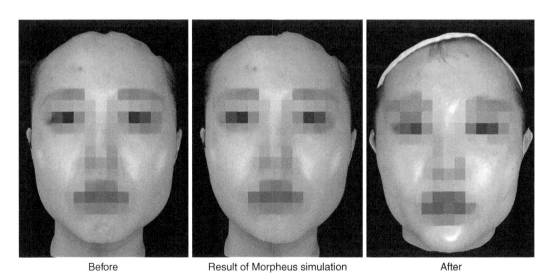

| Before | Result of Morpheus simulation | After |

**Fig. 34.1** Simulation vs actual result of the procedure – front. These are photos of simulation of below the eyes and frontal cheek filler, chin filler, and facial lifting and the actual procedures performed on the same areas

© Springer Nature Singapore Pte Ltd. 2019
B. Kim et al., *The Art and Science of Thread Lifting*, https://doi.org/10.1007/978-981-13-0614-3_34

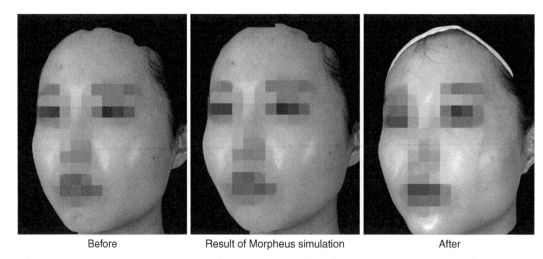

Before                    Result of Morpheus simulation                    After

**Fig. 34.2** Simulation vs result of actual procedure – 45 degrees. These are photos of simulation of below the eyes and frontal cheek filler, chin filler, and facial lifting and the actual procedures performed on the same areas

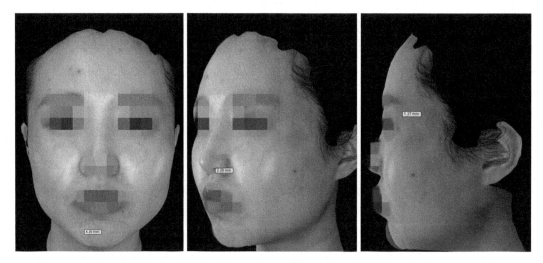

**Fig. 34.3** Simulation of result using Morpheus®. Volume changes after designing using Morpheus system –filler injection simulation to the chin and the frontal cheeks. The areas marked green are areas of increase in volume after simulation. Temple area changes are not by filler but by thread lifting

In such case, the area marked green means the area showing changes in volume in the before and after photos. Namely, the areas newly filled with volume are marked in green.

Based on analysis of the figure, the change in volume of the frontal cheek and the chin areas are results of filler procedures. However, the changes are also observed in temporal area where no insertion procedure was performed. Nonetheless, there was an increase in volume. The reason for this and the production process can be seen in the sequential photos from Fig. 34.4a to f.

### 34.1.3 Interpretation of the Result

Simulation of thread lifting can be done through Morpheus®. At the same time, it is possible to evaluate the outcome of lifting by measuring the volume increase of temporal area.

The volume increase in the green areas can be quantified with Morpheus® system. it is believed that it can be tried for analyzing the outcome of thread lifting in a form different from the GAIS score. This is an area which requires additional researches.

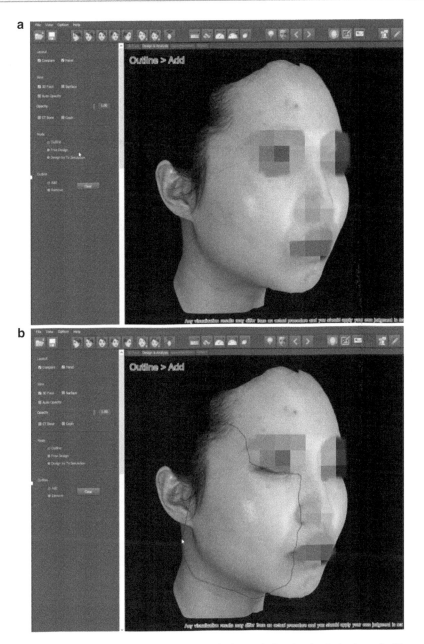

**Fig. 34.4** Simulation using Morpheus®. (**a**) Select a face to perform simulation of lifting. (**b**) Designate the range to apply lifting. (**c**) Perform tasks of moving the facial soft tissues upward within the range. (**d**) Show before and after photos of simulation. (**e**) The area of increased volume before and after the simulation is marked in green. From a different perspective, the size of the increased volume in the green part can be predicted to a certain extent. (**f**) The area of increased volume before and after the simulation view from the different direction

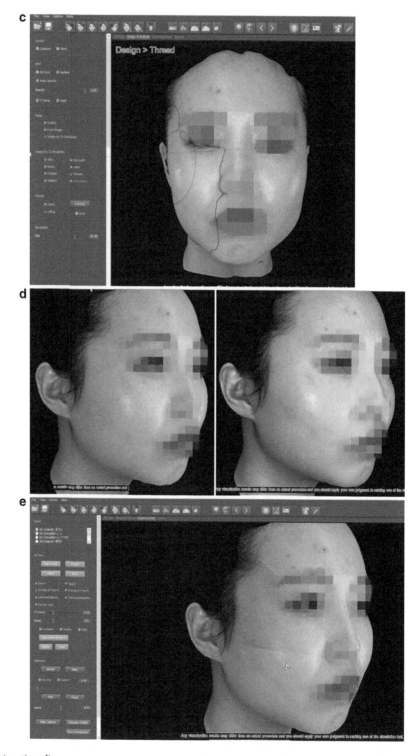

**Fig. 34.4** (continued)

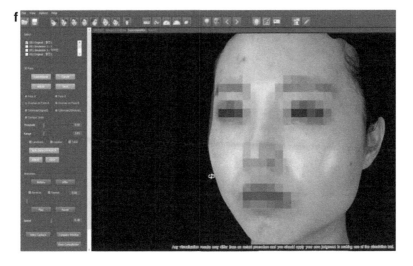

**Fig. 34.4**  (continued)

## 34.2   Evaluation of Before and After Photos Using Morpheus®

As seen in Figs. 34.5 and 34.6, the volume increase in the temporal area due to thread lifting is well presented. It is exactly consistent with the simulation photo by Morpheus®.

If development of technology and physician's know-how are combined, it can be used in objective evaluation tools of thread lifting in the future.

- Simulation of procedure result, catching characteristics such as facial asymmetry, evaluation after the procedure and comparison of before and after, etc. are already being used.
- If AI (=artificial intelligence) system develops more, it is expected that simulation in various forms according to the needs of customers can be developed in the form of real-time showing.

## 34.3   Potential and Future of the Morpheus® System

### 34.3.1  Use

- Morpheus® system would be used in various fields.

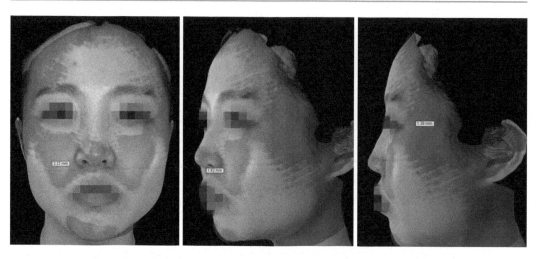

**Fig. 34.5** Evaluation of before and after actual procedure using Morpheus. The area of volume increases after the actual procedure is marked in green. Green area in the frontal hairline and left neck is considered artifact

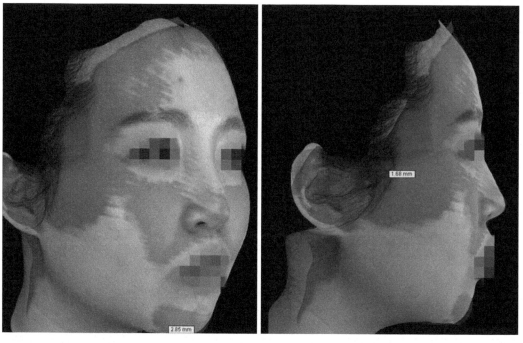

**Fig. 34.6** Evaluation of before and after actual procedure using Morpheus®. Volume increase after the actual procedure (green area). The increased volume in the temporal area is visible. It is exactly consistent with the simulation photos

As it can be seen in the Fig. 35.1, various measurements can be seen utilizing Morpheus. It is possible to assess the change of the patient's face objectively based on numerical data.

Change in volume before and after the procedure can also be known (Fig. 35.2). Volumization can be evaluated after procedures for various areas of the face through color coding.

The Fig. 35.3 shows changes in contour for a specific sagittal and (axial) transverse cross section.

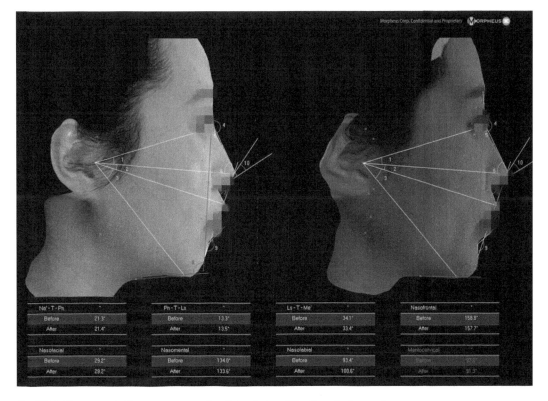

**Fig. 35.1** Easy consultation – measure angle at lateral view. After the actual procedure

© Springer Nature Singapore Pte Ltd. 2019

B. Kim et al., *The Art and Science of Thread Lifting*, https://doi.org/10.1007/978-981-13-0614-3_35

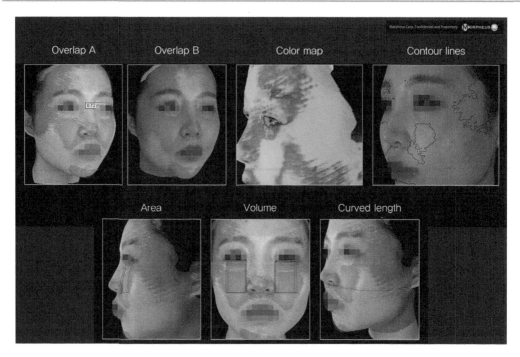

**Fig. 35.2** Easy consultation – evaluation. Based on actual before and after procedure photos, various measurements can be calculated. Through colors, these measurements can be visualized

**Fig. 35.3** Cross section. Prior to the procedure: after Morpheus designing

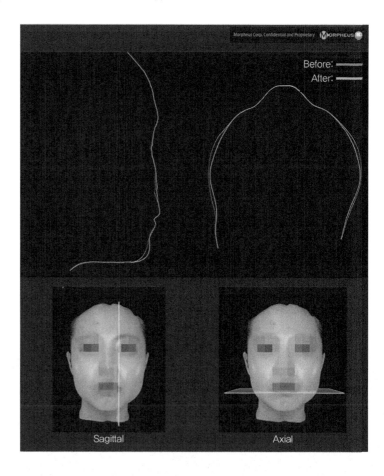

There is a saying that "without experiencing various kinds of side effects, do not say that you know the procedure."

Side effects after procedures are experienced by anyone who has performed procedures. The more the clinical experiences, the higher the likelihood of experiencing side effects. When physicians experience side effects, their relationship with the patient deteriorates and they sometimes experience despair. In some cases, they give up the procedure. The authors have experienced side effects of thread lifting procedures consecutively at some point and were concerned for a long time.

Although there are various types of side effects of thread lifting, there is no side effect as serious as vascular complication of filler. Even if side effects occur in thread lifting, in most cases, they are solved with simple treatments. We would like to introduce the side effects prevention technique and the coping method which have been acquired through the clinical experience, sincerely hoping that our readers will be free from despair and worries from side effects.

# Dissatisfaction

36

The most common complaints related to thread lifting procedures are that the effects are not meeting the patient's expectations. Especially, when procedures are done using threads without cog or short threads with cogs, dissatisfaction occurs a lot. However, due to the development of threads produced using upgraded manufacturing methods recently and techniques, satisfaction level of patients has been much improved.

To reduce dissatisfaction of the effects after the procedure, it is important to help patient set realistic goals and expectations based on the types and number of threads and the condition of the patient's face. Also, satisfaction increases only if patient's expectations are similar to the result of the procedure. Only if overall satisfaction level of thread lifting increases, thread lifting can become more popular and grow further.

The reason for the dissatisfaction after thread lifting can be classified into four categories. This is a subjective categorization by the authors, but if they are categorized prior to approaching them, it helps with post-conditioning.

- Unrealistic expectation of patients
- Patients with challenging facial features
- Outcome limitation of thread lifting products
- Technique issue of the physician

## 36.1 Unrealistic Expectation of Patients

This would probably happen in all cosmetic procedures. If there is a gap between the patient's expectation and the physician's expectation, proper consultation and further communication are required to narrow the gap. The physician has to set realistic and achievable goals to the patient prior to procedure.

## 36.2 Patients for Whom the Procedure Itself Is Difficult

- Depending on the degree of aging and the characteristics of the face, the result of thread lifting varies. Different from surgical treatment, thread lifting does not include the process of removing tissues. Namely, it is a process of rejuvenation through pulling and gathering.
- After consultation, if simulation doesn't ensure good result, surgery may be recommended than noninvasive procedure.

© Springer Nature Singapore Pte Ltd. 2019
B. Kim et al., *The Art and Science of Thread Lifting*, https://doi.org/10.1007/978-981-13-0614-3_36

## 36.3    Structural Limitation of Thread Lifting Products

There are various thread lifting products and mechanism for each. As explained in detail previously, satisfactory results can be obtained based on understanding well the histologic changes from thread insertions in vivo and changes of the appearance following histologic changes. It is impossible to make results that can never be created by the mechanism of a particular product. The suitable product must be chosen based on clearly understanding of mechanisms of each product and comparing the level of objective desired by the physician.

## 36.4    Technique Issues of the Physician

- Whether there is a desired objective, the choice of the right patient group, the right product, and the right technique is important.
- If there is clear understanding of relationship between mechanisms of aging and threads, we can predict that this technique can make satisfactory outcome in advance. Only when the choice of the right product, right technique, and right patient group is made, a desired result can be obtained.

Pains are experienced in some cases after thread lifting procedures.

## 37.1 Points to Verify

- Local or an area
- Accompanying with swelling or not
- Accompanying with fever or not
- Still or making facial expression
- What is felt at palpation: feeling of thread or tissue hanging (whether it is touched strongly differently from other areas)

## 37.2 Cause of Pain

### 37.2.1 Suspected Infection

- This mainly occurs at entry points or areas where threads come out from. All four symptoms, fever, swelling, redness, and pain, occur. If patient's symptom is determined to be related to infection, it is advisable to start treating it as soon as possible.
- As an infection in a special form is related to thread lifting, there is a case of hair getting into the entry point. After observing carefully, if it appears that hair has gotten in, it must be removed. Cautions must be taken not to have it cut during pulling. If the hair is completely buried and is not visible, this generally does not raise any issue, but it can also cause continuous infection in some case.
- In rare cases, although symptom of infection is not clear, the entry point or the exit area continues to swell. Sometimes, although there is no fever or pain, it accompanies fluctuation symptoms.

### 37.2.2 Pain Resulting from Hematoma

If there was severe bleeding and hemostasis was difficult, delayed hematoma may occur. During observation, the swelling area gradually spreads and accompanies bruising. In some cases, swelling is severe in which case the patients suffer. Swelling must be minimized through active compression. As time passes, it naturally calms down. As such it is necessary to ensure the patient.

### 37.2.3 Cog Hanging in a Specific Area

- Dimpling can occur if cog spikes hang strongly in a certain area relatively. This symptom occurs due to inconstant depth during passing a thread, or the cog hangs strongly at the bottom of the dermis near the exit. This situation generally occurs accompanying pain.
- Dimpling from thread lifting is one of the most common side effects, and as patient's

© Springer Nature Singapore Pte Ltd. 2019
B. Kim et al., *The Art and Science of Thread Lifting*, https://doi.org/10.1007/978-981-13-0614-3_37

discomfort is high, it is necessary to solve it as soon as possible.

### 37.2.4 Skin Stimulated by Thread End

- If the thread end is rigid and tapered, in some cases the end area of the thread stimulates the skin. In severe cases, it comes out penetrating through the skin.
- Recently, some leftover threads are made in the form of bending in 180 degrees to make the end soft. This is to prevent the sharp end of the thread from coming out penetrating through the skin.

## 37.3 Treatment According to Cause of Pain

- If infection is suspected → oral antibiotics
- Pain from hematoma → observation and compression
- Cog hanging in a specific area
  - From several days up to 1 month → massage or molding
  - After 1 month → dissection of tangled tissues
- Skin stimulated by thread end → removal of the thread end

When bleeding occurs during the procedure, it is accompanied by bruise, swelling, hematoma, and pain. The causes of bleeding are as follows:

- Damage of the dermal plexus by needle-type thread (sharp cannula)
- Blood vessel damage at the entry point
- Bleeding on the route of cannula insertion

Depending on the types of the threads and technique, the causes of bleeding may differ. Being cautious during the procedure is helpful to prevent bleeding.

## 38.1 Damage of the Dermal Plexus by Needle-Type Thread

When procedures are performed using needle-type thread or sharp cannula, bruise occurs commonly. Even without damages to large blood vessels, as the dermal plexus can be damaged easily, many areas can be bruised.

> **Tip!**
> Even if the procedure is performed using a cannula and if the anesthesia is done using the dental lidocaine prior to the procedure, bruise may occur. To prevent this, using a cannula for anesthesia should be considered.

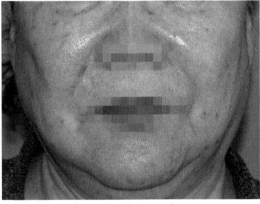 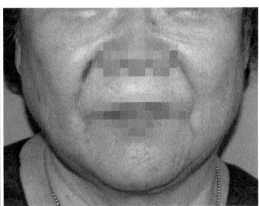

Right after the procedure     One week after the procedure

**Fig. 38.1** Bruise after insertion of needle-type threads (mono PDO threads)

© Springer Nature Singapore Pte Ltd. 2019
B. Kim et al., *The Art and Science of Thread Lifting*, https://doi.org/10.1007/978-981-13-0614-3_38

### 38.1.1  Prevention Method

1. Insert into the subcutaneous layer rather than inserting into the dermis or hypodermis.
2. Insert with a blunt cannula instead of a sharp cannula.

## 38.2  Bleeding at the Entry Point

- This can occur when making an entry point using a sharp needle.
- Especially, it frequently occurs around the hairline or the temporal area. Palpation of the pulse of the artery and careful visual inspection of the vein can be helpful to prevent overlapping the entry point and vessels.
- Superficial temporal artery and vein (STA and STV)
- Sentinel vein (SV)

### 38.2.1  Prevention Method

– Palpation and inspection of vessels during designing.
– SV inspection and STA palpation are better checked at supine position.

**Fig. 38.2** Important blood vessel related to bleeding at entry point – superficial temporal artery. Published with kind permission of © Kwan-Hyun Youn 2018. All rights reserved

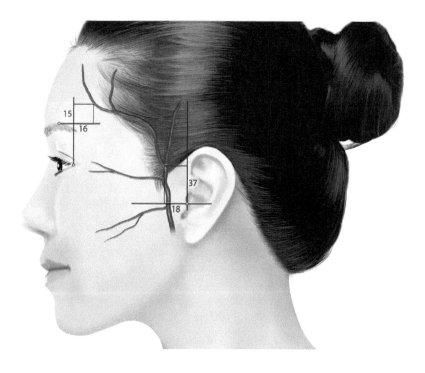

**Fig. 38.3** Important blood vessels related to bleeding of the entry point – tips for designing. (**a**) **Left:** prior to marking the sentinel vein (visible with the naked eye); **Right:** mark the sentinel vein in blue. (**b**) If visual inspection and palpation of blood vessels cannot be done well, perform at supine position or make a bed tilt downward. Blood vessels can be easily observed

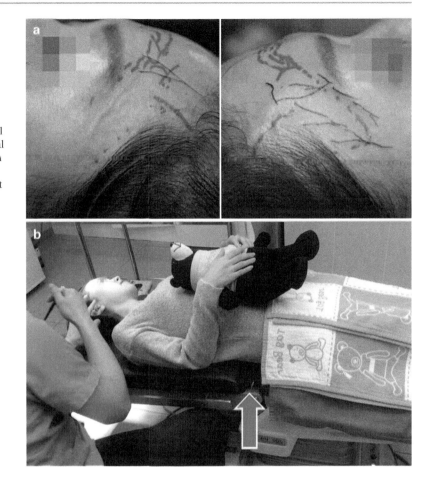

## 38.3   Bleeding on the Route of Cannula Insertion

While inserting a cannula, severe bleeding occurs sometimes. In such case, it is a case of damage in large blood vessels or branches rather than the dermal plexus, and it can develop into hematoma. Especially, in case of insertion with a sharp cannula, the occurrence of bleeding is higher. Also in case of a blunt cannula with a blunt end, caution must be taken as tissue damage and bleeding can sometimes occur in the area where the tissues are dense.

### 38.3.1 Prevention Method

Subcutaneous layer where the blood vessels are sparsely distributed is a proper layer for insertion. The closer it is to the SMAS, the more likely damage occurs to large blood vessels.

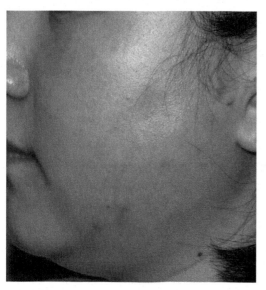

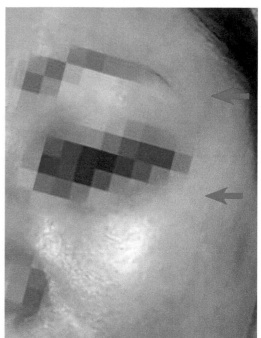

**Fig. 38.4** Bruise and swelling due to bleeding after thread lifting. Damage of the tissues and bleeding around the mouth caused by a sharp cannula

**Summary**

Late Onset Bleeding

A late-onset bruise and swelling can occur a few days later. This rarely happens for procedures using cog threads. This can be caused by blood vessel damage through repetitive stimulation of cogs even if no bleeding occurs during the procedure. Severe bleeding does not occur. Bruise can occur around the orbital area or temporal area accompanied with slight swelling. Under this circumstance, applying compression to the affected area can make symptoms subside.

Within 3–4 days after thread lifting proce-dures, some patients claim that "the threads appear protruded." Although the threads do not actually protrude, a surface of the skin looks elevated along the route of thread insertion while making specific facial expressions (e.g., smiling).

## 39.1 Things to Be Checked Through Examination

- Whether folds are visible with no expression
- Whether it aggravates with facial expressions (especially, when the pronunciation "ee" is made)
- Whether it feels even with palpation

## 39.2 Causes and Solutions

1. When forward/reverse passing of a cannula or needle is overly repeated to insert one thread
   - Minimal swelling occurs along the route of the thread.

**Solution**
   In this case, skin fold is occurred by tempo-rary swelling and generally subsides sponta-neously later.

2. When one of the many threads is pulled by too strong force
   - Especially, if four threads are inserted in each side, this side effect is usually claimed from the fourth (the most medial) thread. This is because the fourth thread passes the area that is closest to the orbital area and the skin in this area is thin.

**Solution**
   1. Increase the number of threads (e.g., 4 → 6).
   2. Pull each thread with the same force.

3. When a thread is inserted into the superficial subcutaneous layer or hypodermis

**Solution**
   Insert thread into a deeper subcutaneous layer

4. When the number of threads is not sufficient to pull the fat tissue
   - When patients have much fat in his/her face, lots of lifting capacity are needed. But this can occur if the number of threads is not enough to hold the weight.

**Solution**
   1. In case of short threads, increase the num-ber of threads.
   2. Insert more short threads additionally between long threads to play a supporting role.

© Springer Nature Singapore Pte Ltd. 2019                                                                                    231
B. Kim et al., *The Art and Science of Thread Lifting*, https://doi.org/10.1007/978-981-13-0614-3_39

After several days or weeks, patients visit the clinic claiming that "the thread is sticking out." The causes of thread protrusion can be categorized as follows:

- Protrusion outside the skin
- Protrusion within the mouth (intraoral)
- Thread near protrusion

In general, this does not accompany infection. It is necessary to check whether the thread is actually sticking out. If removal is necessary, it can be removed with simple measures.

## 40.1   Protrusion Outside the Skin

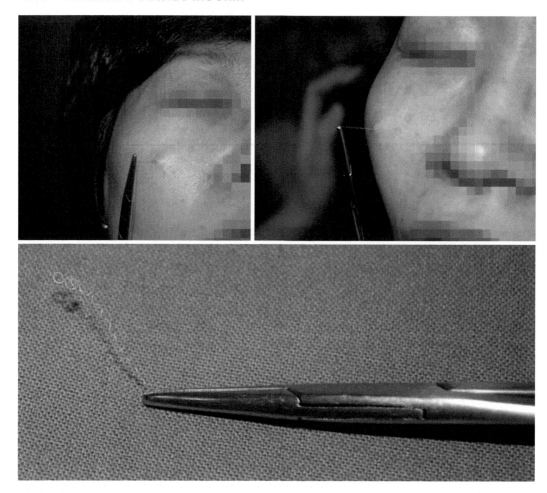

**Fig. 40.1** Protrusion of the thread (outside the skin) and the removed thread. A spiral-type PDO thread was inserted in the frontal cheek. Protrusion of the thread occurred in several days after the procedure. It was removed by pulling the end of the protruded thread with a needle holder

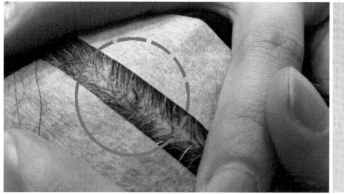

Protruded thread

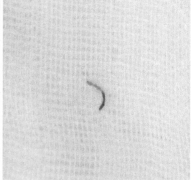

Removed thread

**Fig. 40.2** Protrusion of the thread (outside the skin) and removed thread. A bi-directional PDO cog thread was inserted in the temporal area (see Fig. 6.21). Thread at the entry point was protruded in several days after the procedure. It was removed by pulling the end of the protruded thread with a needle holder

## 40.2 Protrusion Within the Mouth (Intraoral)

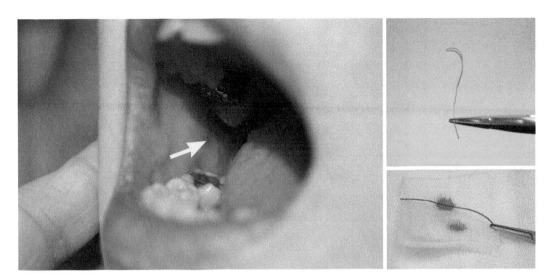

**Fig. 40.3** Protrusion of the thread (intraoral) and removed thread. A bi-directional PDO cog thread was inserted in the lateral cheek. The patient visited clinic claiming pain and protrusion of thread within the mouth in several days (according to the patient, the patient experienced the feeling of the thread being cut while laughing aloud during a meal with friends) Although the thread was cut, the bi-directional part of cog remained, but as the cog was too small and not fixed, it drove downward. It appears to have penetrated the muscle and the oral mucosa. It was removed by pulling the end of the protruded thread with a needle holder

## 40.3   Thread Near Protrusion
## (Impending Protrusion)

**Fig. 40.4** Thread near protrusion (impending protrusion) and removed thread. (**a**) It is more visible while making a facial expression. (**b**) Pushing the skin with the hand makes it more visible. (**c**) The thread is partially cut with scissors holding with a needle holder

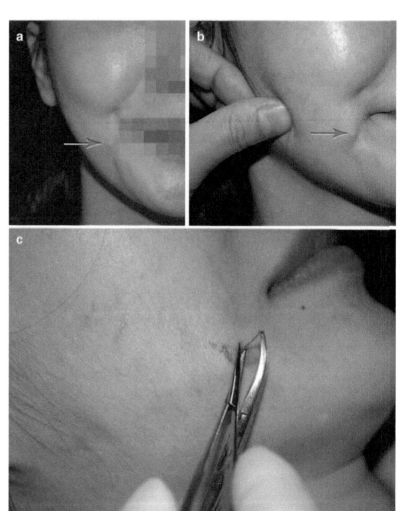

The symptom of migration of threads occurs several weeks after the procedure in general.

Causes of migration are as follows:

- Threads without cog
- Incorrect cutting of bi-directional cog threads
- Breakage of PDO threads due to long-term storage

Patients may complain that the thread has moved or that the thread is likely to come out.

As additional migration can stimulate the skin at the end, it is advisable to remove the thread.

## 41.1 Threads Without Cog

After insertion of the thread without cog, the thread may migrate and be seen through right below the skin. Especially, when it is inserted into around the mouth, which is a dynamic area with facial expressions, sometimes, it can be seen through the thin skin of the jaw line.

## 41.2 Incorrect Cutting of Bi-directional Cog Threads

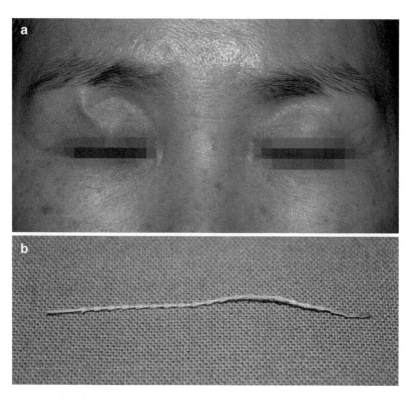

**Fig. 41.1** Thread near protrusion due to migration (after eyebrow lifting) and removed thread. (**a**) A bi-directional PDO cog thread was inserted for eyebrow lifting. Eight weeks after the procedure, the patient claimed "I feel like the thread is about to come out through the eyelid." After stab incision, the thread was entirely removed. The cog should have been inserted in both directions sufficiently from the eyebrow to the hairline, but it was not inserted sufficiently, and the center of the bi-directional cog was cut. Thereafter, the thread which remains only unidirectional cog moved slowly downward and appeared like the above figure (see Fig. 41.2). (**b**) Based on a closer look at the removed thread, as 8 weeks had passed after the procedure, the blue color which was a characteristic of PDO thread disappeared, but it should be noted that the shape of the cog still remained the same

When cutting, cog must be preserved bi-directionally for fixing. Otherwise, if the cutting is done with only unidirectional cog remaining by mistake, it can migrate to one side.

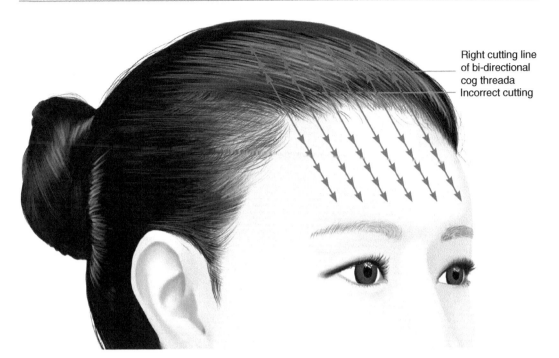

Right cutting line
of bi-directional
cog threada
Incorrect cutting

**Fig. 41.2** Cause of migration of bi-directional cog thread by incorrect cutting. As the reverse directional cogs play a role of fixing point, if all reverse directional cogs are removed, the thread easily moves toward the eyelids. The reverse directional cogs must be kept

## 41.3 Breakage of PDO Threads Due to Long-Term Storage

PDO, which is the key material of thread lifting, easily breaks if exposed to the moisture in the air and cannot restore its strength. Bi-directional cog threads prevent migration through its reverse directional cogs. However, if they are not stored appropriately, these also can be broken into many branches after insertion and migrate.

If too many threads are inserted through one entry point, many ends of threads gather and may look bulging. Even they are cut properly during the process, bulging may occur due to facial expressions. Especially while smiling, as the skin-muscle movement goes superolaterally, the threads migrate to form bulging.

## 42.1 Area of Occurrence

- If an entry point is made at a level where the horizontal line of the lateral canthus and the hairline meet, the likelihood of bulging increases due to zygomaticus muscle movement.
- The likelihood of the occurrence is high if the threads are not appropriately cut.
- In case many thick threads are inserted into one hole (e.g., the likelihood of the occurrence is high when three or four threads of 2-0 thickness are inserted into one hole.)

## 42.2 Solution

- There is no need to cut the threads again by incision if they do not protrude through the skin. As time passes, this gets solved without sequela afterward.

## 42.3 Prevention

- When designing an entry point, check the movement of the skin based on the expression of the zygomaticus muscle.
- Cut appropriately.
- Set an entry point at the eyebrow level or above.

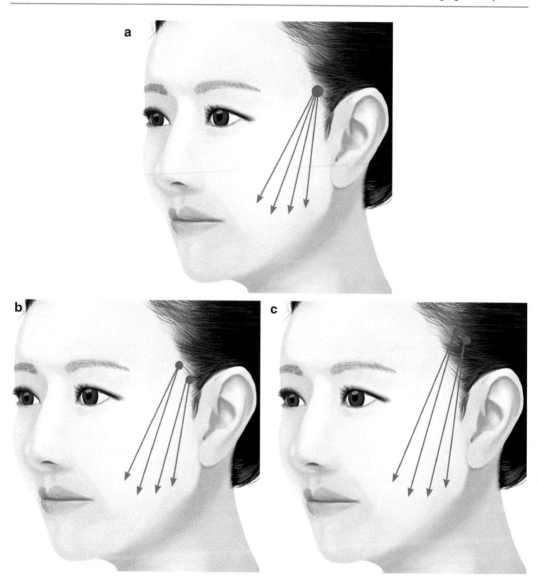

**Fig. 42.1** Occurrence of bulging in relation to number of threads and location of entry point. (**a**) If four threads are inserted into one entry point, the likelihood of occurrence of entry point bulging is high. (**b**) By making two entry points and inserting two threads each, entry point bulging can be prevented. (**c**) If the entry point is located above the hairline not to be exposed, this is a good method for prevention

Most common side effect of cog thread lifting is a depression or a dent in the skin. Especially, it can occur like a dimple in the cheek area.

This can occur right after the procedure or in several days to several weeks after the procedure. This is less likely to occur in general after a month passes.

It sometimes occurs and disappears on its own but a patient claims discomfort and visits the clinic. If physicians do not know how to solve a dimple when they experience this side effect for the first time after thread lifting, it can make them embarrassed. But it improves easily by performing molding using fingers. Depending on the type and insertion area of the thread, the likelihood of occurrence differs. If the likelihood of occurrence and the treatment method after the procedure are explained to the patient prior to treatment, it helps to have a good rapport with the customer.

## 43.1 Mechanism of Dimples Formation

To understand the mechanism of dimples formation after thread lifting procedures, it is necessary to know the difference in density of fibrotic tissues within the fat layer first. The area where cogs hang properly after thread insertion is where a certain amount of fibrotic tissues are dispersed within the fat tissues. In that way, the cog does not slip after lifting and holds in position and it results in good effect.

However, if there are too much fibrotic tissues within the fat tissues, which are too dense, it is difficult for a cannula or a needle to pass. Also, as cogs can fix well in undesired locations rather than their original locations, dimples are formed easily.

© Springer Nature Singapore Pte Ltd. 2019
B. Kim et al., *The Art and Science of Thread Lifting*, https://doi.org/10.1007/978-981-13-0614-3_43

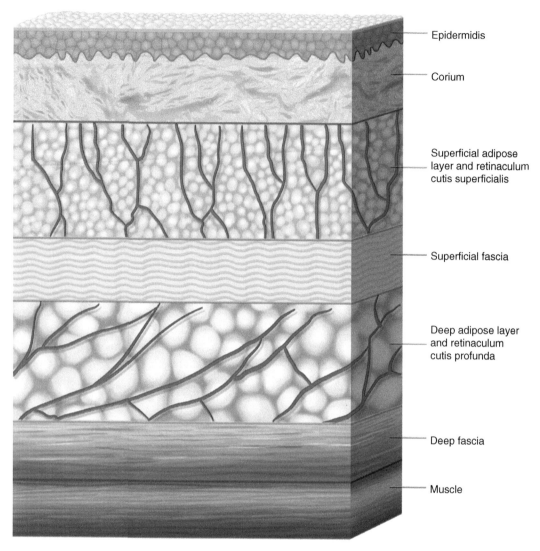

Epidermidis

Corium

Superficial adipose
layer and retinaculum
cutis superficialis

Superficial fascia

Deep adipose layer
and retinaculum
cutis profunda

Deep fascia

Muscle

**Fig. 43.1** Difference in density of fibrotic tissue within the fat tissues in facial areas. Depending on facial area, some fat tissues are divided into superficial fat layer and deep fat layer and some fat tissues have only one fat layer. What is important is the density of fat tissues. Soft fat tissues like cheese can be easily passed by a cannula or needle. But they can't easily pass in dense fat tissue. It is useful for the procedure to understand which area in the face has soft or dense fat tissues (see Fig. 6.69)

### 43.1.1 Inconstant Insertion Depth of Cogs

If a depth of thread insertion is not constant, some cogs hang in the dense hypodermis, and some cogs hang in the loose subcutaneous fat layer, in which dimples can be formed.

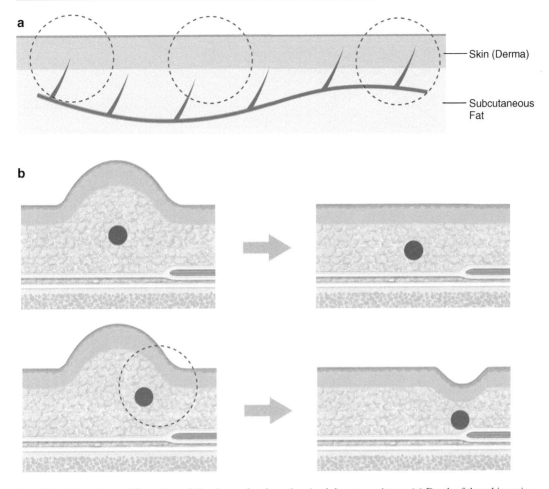

**Fig. 43.2** Mechanisms of formation of dimples – when insertion depth is not consistent. (**a**) Depth of thread insertion is not consistent. (**b**) Dimple from insertion at inconstant depth during pinch technique (cross section)

- Pinch technique is used variously to prevent blood vessel damage and to insert the thread at constant depth. However, if the force of pinch is not adequately controlled, this can cause sinking of the skin.
- Through pinch technique, the subcutaneous fat layer is elevated and insertion with constant depth can be performed. But sometimes sinking can occur unexpectedly. Physicians who have performed liposuction probably have experienced a dent in the skin through the same mechanism.
- As shown in Fig. 43.2b, if the thread does not adequately passed the correct layer, namely, insertion is done from the side rather than the middle part of the pinch, sinking can occur.

### 43.1.2  Sinking of Cutting Parts

In some thread lifting technique, the end of the thread should be cut and buried sufficiently within the fat layer. But if the buried cogs hang in dermis layer or dense fibrotic tissues of fat layer, sinking can occur.

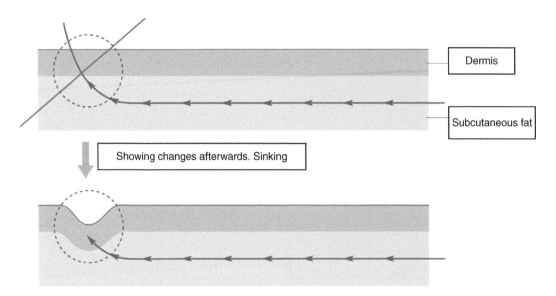

**Fig. 43.3** Mechanisms of formation of dimples – sinking of cutting parts. The last part of the cut thread must be sufficiently buried in to the subcutaneous layer. Sinking occurs if it hangs in the bottom part of the dermis

### 43.1.3  When Some Cogs Are Not Hung Consistently in the Dermal Layer

The pink circled dotted line in Fig. 43.4 shows the area where cogs hang in the dermis. When a thread with strong cogs hangs partially in the dermis or hypodermis inconsistently, the skin where the cogs hang strongly can be sunken.

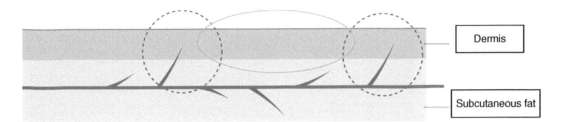

**Fig. 43.4**  Mechanisms of formation of dimples

## 43.2   Type of Dimples Depending on Area

### 43.2.1   Dimples in the Route of Thread Insertion

**Fig. 43.5** Causes of dimples – dimples in the route of thread insertion. (**a**) Insertion method without exit points. (**b**) Temporal anchoring method

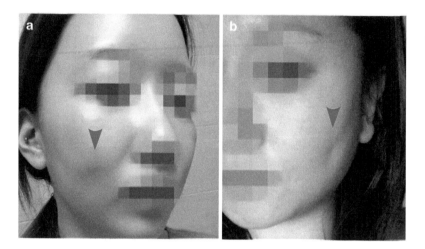

**Fig. 43.6** Area of occurrence. It frequently occurs where the subcutaneous fat tissues are too fibrotic or where change of facial expression results in excessive motion of muscle (elliptical area in orange – near the oral angle)

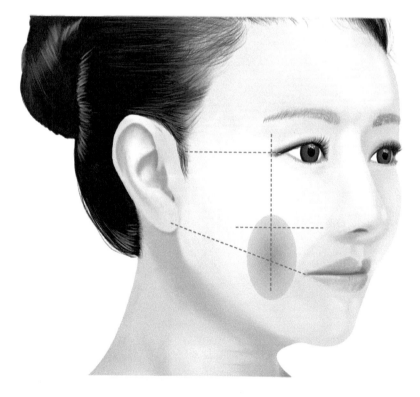

1. Management of dimples (in case of dimples in Rt. side).
   ① Put on a glove on the Lt. hand and lay the index finger on the inner side of the dimple in oral cavity.
   ② Position the index finger of the Rt. hand right on the dimple, and push the skin downward giving snaps in the direction of the extended line of the thread insertion.
   ③ It is untangled with a feeling of clicking and the cog hangs at the original location.
2. When dimples suddenly occur after excessive motion of facial muscles
   Sometimes dimples do not occur after the procedure but can appear later after laughing aloud or eating food with the mouth wide open.
   ① **Cause**
      Due to change in the facial expressions (esp, contraction of the zygomaticus muscle), dimples are formed suddenly while the tissues where the thread is inserted move with the muscle motion, and the cog is fixed at a new location (about 2–5 mm, superior-lateral) other than the original location.
   ② **Area of occurrence**
      The area within approximately 2FB (finger breadth) distant from the oral angle and where the subcutaneous tissues are very fibrotic, dimples are easily formed through changes in facial expressions.

③ **Solution**
   (a) Put on a glove on the Lt. hand and lay the index finger on the inner side of the dimple in oral cavity.
   (b) Position the index finger of the Rt. hand right on the dimple and push the skin downward                giving                snaps inferomedially.
   (c) It is untangled with a feeling of clicking and the cog hangs at the original location.
④ **Progress**
   • Dimples usually form within 1 to 2 weeks after the procedure rather than right after the procedure.
   • It rarely occurs after a month.
   • This can recur at home even after solving by maneuver with fingers in clinic. Accordingly, by showing the maneuver with fingers in a mirror, it can be solved by oneself when it recurs at home.
   • It is recommended that physicians provide explanations about the likelihood of dimples and easy solutions prior to the procedure.
3. Prevention of dimples
   When inserting a thread into the medial side of the face, the likelihood of dimples increases if the thread is inserted up to the area close to the oral angle. If the threads in ③ and in ④ (Fig. 43.7) are inserted up to the blue line, rather than going up to the elliptical area in orange, dimples resulting from facial expressions can be prevented.

**Fig. 43.7** Prevention of dimples

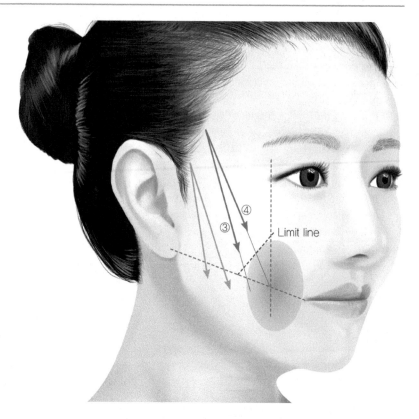

## 43.2.2 Dimple at Exit Point (U Technique: Anchoring Method)

This is the case right after cutting the thread at the exit point, which is the last stage of the procedure (Fig. 43.8).

The mechanism is illustrated in Fig. 43.3.

However, it flattens simply by pushing the skin while giving snaps with the fingers. In some cases, dimples form in the exit point in several days after the procedure like in Fig. 43.5. In such case, it can be solved by the same method as managing dimples in the route of thread insertion.

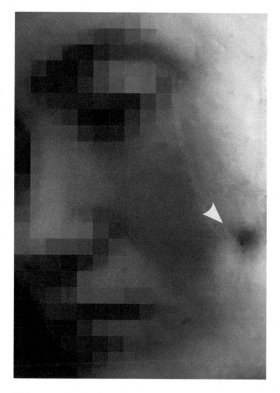

**Fig. 43.8** Cause of dimple – dimple at exit point

### 43.2.3 Dimple at Entry Point (U Technique: Anchoring Method)

#### 43.2.3.1 Mechanisms of Formation of the Entry Point Dimple

- Basically, as thread lifting is a method of pulling sagging skin, some areas are slightly folded or wrinkled. As the pulled skin is not gone, if the bottom part is pulled upward, a dimple can naturally occur to a certain extent at the entry point.
- A fixing point is formed laterally to the hairline. Therefore, even if some skin is folded, entry point dimple is rarely exposed as entry point lies on the scalp.
- However, as a severe dimple which forms in the entry point occurs due to inappropriate technique, a delicate skill is needed while lifting with temporal fascia anchoring.

**Summary**

Distinguishing entry point dimples – normal dimple vs side effects

When both ends of the thread are slightly pulled using one hand while the thread is inserted from the entry point to the exit point in a U shape:

- If dimple forms → incorrect procedure
- If no dimple forms → normal

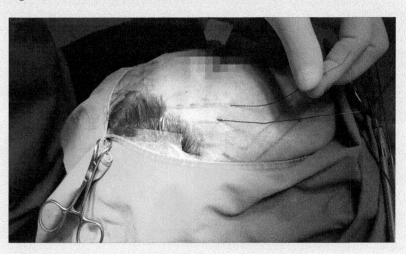

### 43.2.3.2 Prevention of Entry Point Dimple

- Make an appropriate size of hole for an entry point.
- Make a route for easy passing for the thread to pass easily in a U shape.
- Especially, it is necessary for the thread not to hang in the bottom of the dermis at each entry point (Fig. 43.9).

### 43.2.3.3 Treatment

① Dissection using scissors

Dissect the space between the dermis and the subcutaneous fat using scissors with sharp ends.

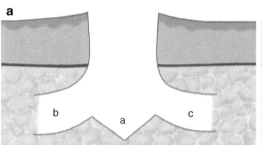 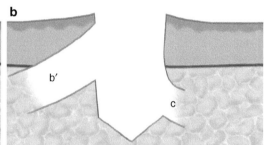

**Fig. 43.9** Causes and prevention of entry point dimple. (**a**) In making an entry point, after puncturing a hole (a) perpendicularly, make a passage in both directions. Once the thread is inserted at a constant depth within the subcutaneous fat from b-a-c, a dimple does not form even if the thread is pulled. (**b**) In case of making inappropriate size of holes for an entry point or inserting the thread through a new hole due to incorrect passage of a cannula/needle rather than ready-made hole, a dimple forms if the thread is pulled

# Sunken Cheek

There is an area where the cheek is slightly hollow on the side of the face. This is called "sunken cheek," which is considered to make a charming face in Western country. However, Asian women tend not to like this. Sunken cheek is not noticeable in some young patients, but it stands out more as they grow older.

Sometimes patients who originally had sunken cheeks complain that the cheek sunk after lifting procedure. Or they claim there is asymmetry between the left and the right. These can happen if the physicians did not confirm to the patients prior to the procedure.

Only when the physicians are aware of the cause and clinical meaning of the sunken cheek prior to the procedure, claims of patients after the procedure can be avoided.

## 44.1 Anatomical Structure

- It is a structure consisting of the zygomatic-cutaneous ligament and masseteric-cutaneous ligament (Fig. 44.1).
- The location on the cheek and the angle of sagging differ between individuals.

© Springer Nature Singapore Pte Ltd. 2019
B. Kim et al., *The Art and Science of Thread Lifting*, https://doi.org/10.1007/978-981-13-0614-3_44

**Fig. 44.1** Marking the sunken cheek area. (**a**) Normal state. (**b**) If the skin on the zygomatic arch is lifted, it goes up well (upward vector). (**c**) If the skin on the zygomatic arch is pushed downward, it does not go down well but moves toward inside (inward vector). (**d**) Using a pen, mark the sunken cheek area in a triangle or a diamond shape

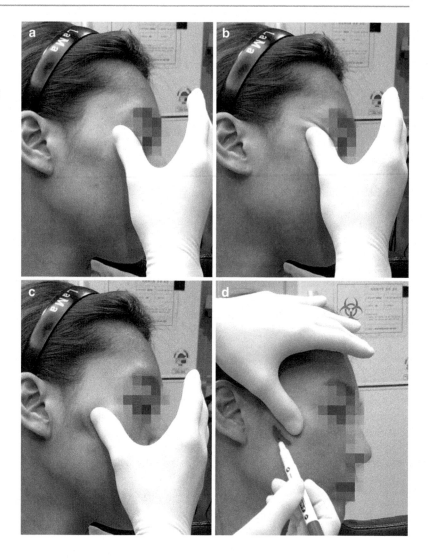

**Fig. 44.2** Sunken cheek. Sunken cheek is noticeable in older patients. As it is an area of severe skin adhesion, cautions must be taken during thread lifting procedures

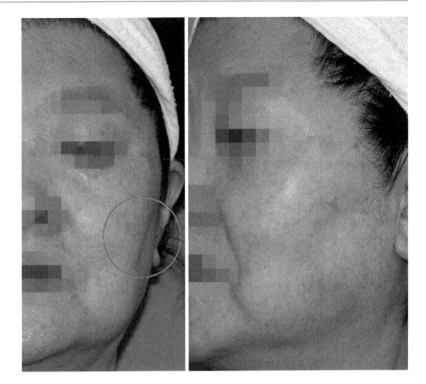

## 44.2    Clinical Importance

- If the skin is pushed inferior-laterally with the hand, significant feature can be observed. When the skin of other facial parts is pushed upward/downward with fingers, the skin is moved in accordance with the direction of the fingers upward/downward. However, when the skin on sunken cheek is pushed superomedially, it is moved in the same direction, but if it is moved inferolaterally, it can be observed that the skin is folded inward (namely, the inner vector affects). The skin of other facial parts is moved in the direction of the fingers in upward/downward vector, this area is affected by upward/inner vector (Fig. 44.2).

- As this area has little fat and consists of ligaments and fibrotic tissues, it is hard to pass during the procedure. Moreover, once cogs hang here, they are fixed and nearly at standstill. As a result, sinking occurs even further after the procedure.

## 44.3    Cautions

- Confirm to patients whether there is a sunken cheek prior to the procedure.
- Check if there is any difference between the right and the left sides prior to the procedure.
- Explain that even the lower cheek is lifted well this area may not be resolved well.

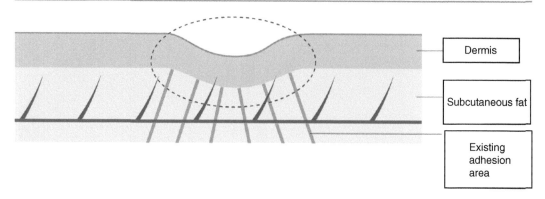

**Fig. 44.3** Cause of dimple – when cogs hang in the area of severe adhesion. Green line indicates existing adhesion → the skin is sunk originally. The interval between cogs (blue) is consistent. Nonetheless, as some cogs hang in fibrotic and dense area (red dotted line), the existing sinking aggravates

# Temporary Paralysis of the Facial Nerves

In some cases, patients and physicians both become surprised by the asymmetrical facial expressions after the procedure. Especially, they discover that when the patients attempt to look in the mirror with eyes open, the eyebrows do not elevate well or asymmetry shows in facial expressions. Sometimes it could be unilateral or bilateral.

## 45.1 Cause

If local anesthetic agent is injected for pain control, this could anesthetize not only the sensory nerves but also motor nerves. It is unlikely that a cannula would damage to motor nerves which is located in the space between the SMAS and the muscle. However, due to the diffusion of lidocaine, motor nerves can be anesthetized.

## 45.2 Clinical Features

- "It is hard to close the eyes" (anesthesia of the orbicularis oculi muscle) → Paralysis of the zygomatic branch due to anesthesia of the zygomatic arch

- "It is hard to open the eyes" (anesthesia of the frontalis muscle) → Paralysis of the frontal branch due to anesthesia of the temple
- "The mouth turns" (anesthesia of the zygomaticus major/minor muscle) → Paralysis of the buccal branch due to anesthesia of the side cheek
- In most cases, the patients confirm this while looking in the mirror right after the procedure, but sometimes they recognize after going back home (in 2–3 h after the procedure). This is the case that they do not check thoroughly right after the procedure and find out after looking in the mirror closely at home.

## 45.3 Solution

- Reassurance.
- If the procedure is performed in the afternoon, it usually recovers by the evening or before going to sleep at night. Sometimes, the symptom remains until the dawn and restores in the morning.

**Summary**

When local anesthesia for thread lifting and botulinum toxin treatment on forehead are performed simultaneously

If various procedures are performed at the same time, usually, the long procedure is done first and the simple procedure is done lastly. Botulinum toxin treatment on the forehead needs to set injection points while moving the frontalis muscle and the eyebrows. But if the frontalis muscle is temporarily paralyzed after the thread lifting, it is difficult to set the injection point on the forehead. Therefore, it is advisable to treat the botulinum toxin first in the muscle areas where temporary paralysis can occur and then perform the thread lifting thereafter.

Elevation of the lateral canthus after the procedure can be obtained only when outstanding techniques are used. Usually, this effect could be achieved with temporal anchoring method. But many patients tend to claim that they look fierce after the procedure due to this effect.

## 46.1 Cause

In Fig. 46.1, it can occur when the distance between the fourth thread and the lateral canthus is shorter than about 2FB.

## 46.2 Solution

- Set an entry point to make at least 2FB in distance between the fourth thread and the lateral canthus.

- Do not pull too strongly during traction of the fourth thread (use an even and firm pulling).

## 46.3 Prevention

- During designing prior to the procedure, it must be explained to the patients that the lateral canthus may be elevated after the procedure.
- Although the lateral canthus can be elevated slightly immediately after the procedure, when the swelling is released within 2–3 days, it restores to normal. However, as some patients could overreact to the elevation of the lateral canthus, caution must be taken.

B. Kim et al., *The Art and Science of Thread Lifting*, https://doi.org/10.1007/978-981-13-0614-3_46

**Fig. 46.1** Cause and prevention of lateral canthus elevation

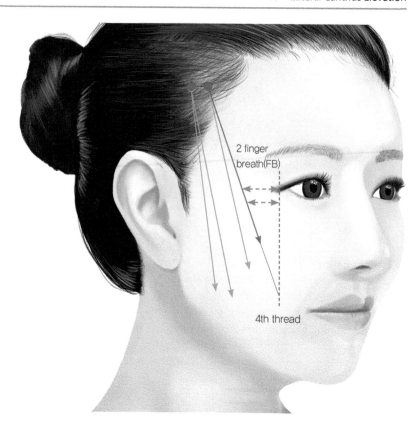

**Summary**
Utilization of lateral canthus elevation

- Some young patients desire elevation of the lateral canthus. For these patients, by designing location of the fourth thread properly, satisfactory result can be increased.

- Even for middle-aged patients who are concerned with dropping of the lateral canthus or the eyebrows, if the lateral canthus is slightly elevated by thread lifting, it can be utilized as a procedure for periorbital rejuvenation.

## 47.1 Thread Lifting and Infection

According to Park TH et al., when nonabsorbable thread lifting was mainly used in the past, cases of chronic inflammation like foreign body granuloma as well as infection occurred in low incidence.

Wu et al. discussed that infection or granuloma formation can occur during thread lifting procedure. However, fortunately, the most complications such as infection are not severe and can be treated easily. However, Benny Yau et al. reported a case of Mycobacterium abscessus infection after performing a thread lifting procedure on the face. It is an important case which shows severe infection can occur although it is rare.

Infection after absorbable thread lifting is evaluated to be less frequent than infections after nonabsorbable thread lifting. If the operating room maintains good hygiene, infection on the thread insertion area does not occur easily.

Also, in case of the PDO (polydioxanone) which is used the most in absorbable thread lifting, it can be manufactured with smooth surface and in the form of monofilament. Therefore, it tends to have higher resistance against infection relatively.

However, recently, cases of mycobacterium infections were reported after PDO thread lifting procedures in Korea. Shin Jung Jin et al. reported a case of a 47-year-old woman who came in with erythematous plaque on both sides which occurred in the second week after the procedure from a nonmedical practitioner. The patient was treated with antibiotics for 1 week at a local clinic and transferred to general hospital, and it was finally diagnosed as *Mycobacterium massiliense* infection.

Therefore, medical practitioners should keep in mind all possibilities of infections and try to maintain a sterile environment before and after procedures.

## 47.2 Prevention of Infections

To prevent infections, areas around entry points must be disinfected thoroughly, and aseptic technique should be used during the procedure.

- Disinfect entry points.
- Disinfect all of the skin area within the range of cannula manipulation.
- If there is hair within the access of cannula or if insertion is done inside the scalp, hair must be prepared using suitable tools.
- Hair must not be dragged into the entry points during the procedure.
- After the procedure, check once more whether any hair got in the entry points.
- Education for prevention of infections at the entry points and the exits.

© Springer Nature Singapore Pte Ltd. 2019
B. Kim et al., *The Art and Science of Thread Lifting*, https://doi.org/10.1007/978-981-13-0614-3_47

## 47.3    Treatment

Infection after thread lifting procedure is generally treated easily by taking antibiotics. However, in rare cases, as mentioned above, mycobacterium infection needs a long-term treatment with intravenous antibiotics and drainage process.

In case of infection which is irresponsive to antibiotics treatment, transferring a patient to the general hospital must be considered and aggressive treatment is required.

In the case of *Mycobacterium massiliense* infection, as mentioned above, a long-term treatment with clarithromycin and amikacin was done after drainage.

# Appendices

## 1.1    Appendix 1: Summary

*Summary*

### PART 03   Why Pinch Anatomy?

*Summary*

### PART 05    Basic Techniques

© Springer Nature Singapore Pte Ltd. 2019
B. Kim et al., *The Art and Science of Thread Lifting*, https://doi.org/10.1007/978-981-13-0614-3

*Summary*

*Summary*

Summary

## PART 07  Procedures for Each Area

Summary

## PART 09  Side Effects and Treatments

## 1.2 Appendix 2: Procedure Records

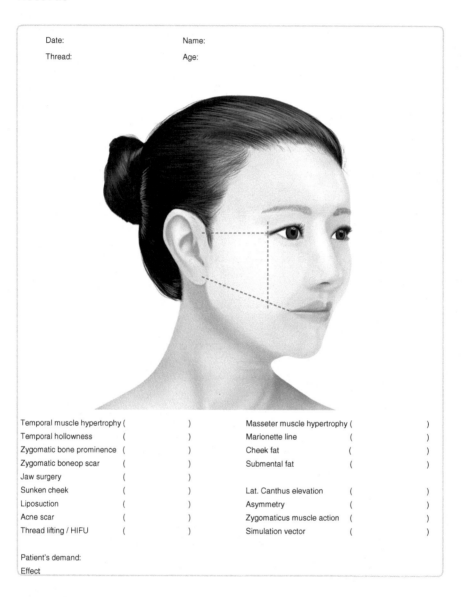

Date:                              Name:

Thread:                           Age:

| | | | | |
|---|---|---|---|---|
| Temporal muscle hypertrophy ( | ) | Masseter muscle hypertrophy ( | ) |
| Temporal hollowness ( | ) | Marionette line ( | ) |
| Zygomatic bone prominence ( | ) | Cheek fat ( | ) |
| Zygomatic boneop scar ( | ) | Submental fat ( | ) |
| Jaw surgery ( | ) | | |
| Sunken cheek ( | ) | Lat. Canthus elevation ( | ) |
| Liposuction ( | ) | Asymmetry ( | ) |
| Acne scar ( | ) | Zygomaticus muscle action ( | ) |
| Thread lifting / HIFU ( | ) | Simulation vector ( | ) |

Patient's demand:

Effect

## Further Readings

Abraham RF, et al. Thread-lift for facial rejuvenation: assessment of long-term results. Arch Facial Plast Surg. 2009;11(3):178–83.

Agarwal CA, et al. The course of the frontal branch of the facial nerve in relation to fascial planes: an anatomic study. Plast Reconstr Surg. 2010;125:532–7.

Amuso D, et al. Histological evaluation of a biorevitalisation treatment with PDO wires. Aesthetic Medicine 13 October–December 2015.

Atiyeh BS, et al. Barbed sutures "lunch time" lifting: evidence-based efficacy. J Cosmet Dermatol. 2010;9:132–41.

Beer K. Delayed complications from thread-lifting: report of a case, discussion of treatment options, and consideration of implications for future technology. Dermatol Surg. 2008;34:1120–3.

Bergerer-Galley C. Comparison of resorbable soft tissue fillers. Aesthet Surg J. 2004;24:33–46.

Carron MA, et al. Biochemical analysis of anchoring points in Rhitidectomy. Arch Facial Plast Surg. 2010;12(1):37–9.

De Carolis V, Gonzalez M. Neck rejuvenation with mastoid-spanning barbed tensor threads (MST operation). Aesth Plast Surg. 2014;38(3):491–500. https://doi.org/10.1007/s00266-014-0288-4.

DeLorenzi CL. Barbed sutures: rationale and technique. Aesthetic Surg J. 2006;26:223–9.

Donath AS, et al. Volume loss versus gravity: new concepts in facial ageing. Curr Opin Otolaryngol Head Neck Surg. 2007;15:238–43.

Fisher GL, et al, Looking older: fibroblast collapse and therapeutic implications. Arch Dermatol. 2008;144:666–72.

Fitzgerald R, et al. Nonsurgical modalities to treat the aging face. Aesthetic Surg J. 2010;30(Suppl):31s–5s.

Goldberg D, et al. Single arm study for the characterization of human tissue response to injectable poly-L-lactic acid. Dermatol Surg. 2013;1–8.

Han HH, et al. Combined, minimally invasive, thread-based facelift. Arch Aesthetic Plast Surg. 2014;20(3):160–4.

Hartmann D, et al. Complications associated with cutaneous aesthetic procedures. J Dtsch Dermatol Ges. 2015;13:778–86. https://doi.org/10.1111/ddg.12757.

Jackson JL, et al. Botulinum toxin a for prophylactic treatment of migraine and tension headache in adults a meta-analysis. JAMA. 2012;307(16):1736–45. https://doi.org/10.1001/jama.2012.505.

Jung WS, et al. Clinical implications of the middle temporal vein with regard to temporal fossa augmentation. Dermatol Surg. 2014 Jun;40(6):618–23.

Kim H, et al. Novel Polydioxanone multifilament scaffold device for tissue regeneration. Dermatol Surg. 2016;42:63–7.

Kurita M, et al. Tissue reactions to cog structure and pure gold in lifting threads: a histological study in rats. Aesthet Surg J. 2011;31(3):347–51.

Lee Y, Hwang K. Skin thickness of Korean adults. Surg Radiol Anat. 2002;24:183–9.

Lee JG, et al. Frontal branch of the superficial temporal artery: anatomical study and clinical implications regarding injectable treatments. Surg Radiol Anat. 2015;37:61–8.

Mendelson B, Wong CH. Changes in the facial skeleton with aging: implications and clinical applications in facial rejuvenation. Aesthet Plast Surg. 2012;36:753–60.

Mendelson B, Wong CH. Anatomy of the aging face. In: Neligan PC, editor. Plastic surgery. 3rd ed. Philadelphia: Elsevier Saunders; 2013. p. 78–92.

Park TH, et al. The efficacy of peri-lesional surgical approach for foreign body granuloma. Plast Reconstr Surg. 2011;127:121–3.

Paul MD. Barbed sutures in aesthetic plastic surgery: evolution of thought and process. Aesthet Surg J. 2013;33(3S):17S–31S.

Prendergast P. Minimally invasive face and neck lift using silhouette coned sutures. In: Miniinvasive face and body lifts – closed suture lifts or barbed thread lifts. https://doi.org/10.5772/51677.

Rachel JD, et al. Incidence of complications and early recurrence in 29 patients after facial rejuvenation with barbed suture lifting. Dermatol Surg. 2010;36:348–54.

Ruff G. Technique and uses for absorbable barbed sutures. Aesthet Surg J. 2006;26:620–8.

Ruff GL. The history of barbed sutures. Aesthet Surg J. 2013;33(3S):12S–6S.

Sapountzis S, et al. Successful treatment of thread-lifting complication from APTOS sutures using a simple MACS lift and fat grafting. Aesthetic Plast Surg. 2012;36:1307–10.

Savoia A, Accardo C, Vannini F, et al. Outcomes in thread lift for facial rejuvenation: a study performed with happy lift revitalizing. Dermatol Ther (Heidelb). 2014 Jun;4(1):103–14.

Shin JJ, et al. *Mycobacterium massiliense* infection after thread-lift insertion. Dermatol Surg. 2016;42(10):1219–22.

Suh DH, et al. Outcomes of polydioxane knotless thread lifting for facial rejuvenation. Dermatol Surg. 2015;41:720–5.

Sulamanidze M, Sulamanidze G. APTOS suture lifting methods: 10 years of experience. Clin Plast Surg. 2009;36:281–306.

Sulamanidze M, et al. Avoiding complications with Aptos sutures. Aesthet Surg J. 2011;31(8):863–73.

Tabira Y, et al. Superficial Musculoaponeurotic system and the facial soft tissues. In: Watanabe K, et al., editors. Anatomy for plastic surgery of the face, head, and neck: thieme; 2016. p. 101–10.

Tajirian AL, Goldberg DJ. A review of sutures and other skin closure materials. J Cosmet Laser Ther. 2010;12:296–302.

Watson S-W, Morales-Ryan C-A, Sinn D-P. Poster 14: internal midface lift: the foundation for facial rejuvenation. J Oral Maxillofac Surg. 2003;61(8S1):88.

Winkler E, et al. Stensen duct rupture (Sialocele) and other complications of the Aptos thread technique. Plast Reconstr Surg. 2006;118:1468.

Wu WTL. Barbed sutures in facial rejuvenation. Aesthet Surg J. 2004;24:582–7.

Yang HM, et al. Sihler staining study of anastomosis between the facial and trigeminal nerves in the ocular area and its clinical implications. Muscle Nerve. 2013;48:545–50.

Yang H-M, et al. Anatomical study of medial zygomaticotemporal vein and its clinical implication regarding the injectable treatments. Surg Radiol Anat. 2015;37:175–80.

Yau B, et al. *Mycobacterium abscessus* abscess post-thread facial rejuvenation procedure. www.ePlasty.com. Interesting Case, April 7, 2015.

Yoo KH, et al. Chronic inflammatory reaction after thread lifting: delayed unusual complication of nonabsorbable thread. Dermatol Surg. 2015;41(4):510–3.

Yoon JH, et al. Tissue changes over time after polydioxanone thread insertion: an animal study with pigs. J Cosmet Dermatol. https://doi.org/10.1111/jocd.12718.

Printed by Printforce, the Netherlands